About the Author

Martina Tierney is an Author, Educator and Clinical Director at Seating Matters, the company she founded to help achieve her goal of transforming healthcare through appropriate seating. Martina is also Clinical Director at A1 Risk Solutions, an expert Moving and Handling business in the UK acquired in 2024. More than anything though, Martina is a passionate Occupational Therapist (OT).

Throughout her 40-year career, she has worked in acute and community care, nursing homes and rehabilitation. She has studied the benefits of postural support and has designed clinical seating which continues to transform the lives of patients around the world daily.

Acknowledgements

Writing a book is not a solo job. It takes a team, and I am very fortunate to have that team inhouse.

My appreciation goes to Dearbhaile Mulholland for all the editing, proofreading and helpful suggestions she made in the completion of this book in a very tight time frame. She spent countless hours at home and in the office to get it just right. She is a true professional.

I am indebted to Gary Boyd who is a creative and talented artist responsible for the book design and layout. Gary's attention to detail is evident in the front cover design, the illustrations and the layout which has greatly enhanced the message of the book.

Finally, I am very grateful to my son Jonathan who has been a huge inspiration and encourager of this book. He was enthusiastic from the start and has made many helpful suggestions which have added to the power of the book. He has read it many times to reassure and boost my confidence when I needed it. I give him credit for the title of the book.

I would like to dedicate this book to all
the contributors who told their story.
Your contribution has enhanced the book
immensely and made it a delightful gift to the
OT world and beyond.

I would also like to dedicate it to all the
Occupational Therapists past and present who
have transformed the lives of so many people
by your dedication, commitment and care.

Martina Tierney

Contents

Continued...

Part II - In conversation with...

The

POWER

of

OT

Heartfelt Stories from
Occupational Therapists

Martina Tierney

"It's not enough to give a patient something to do with their hands. You must reach for the heart as well as the hands. It's the heart that really does the healing."

Ora Ruggles,
A pioneer in Occupational Therapy

Foreword

by
Professor Katrina Bannigan

This book is long overdue. I recommend it to everyone working in the Occupational Therapy profession—students, new graduates, specialists, team or service leads, academics—or anyone considering becoming an Occupational Therapist. It has been written for you. That it exists at all is the mark of its author Martina Tierney, she is an extraordinary Occupational Therapist, who founded Seating Matters; an international business that provides therapeutic seating to people across the world. In her story she provides an honest account of how Seating Matters came into being and, in doing so, shows that she is the living embodiment of the power of occupation to change lives. She pulls back the curtain to explain how she moved from working in the community to setting up Seating Matters. Martina is nearing the end of her career but, in writing this book, she is still contributing at the highest level and making a difference. We can all learn from her powerful story to move our profession forward.

The Power of Occupational Therapy

Martina recognises that Occupational Therapists are responsible for how Occupational Therapy is understood. Her motivation in writing the book is to share uplifting stories about how Occupational Therapists transform lives. To this end, the central theme of the book is the Power of Occupational Therapy as a force for good, for the people and communities we work with, for us, as Occupational Therapists, and for society. The power of occupation is elucidated through Martina's own story but, although she is the driving force behind the book, the book is not just about her. She has also included a series of interviews with other Occupational Therapists who have inspired her. In these interviews she has, like I did in the RCOT* Elizabeth Casson Memorial Lecture 2024, identified Occupational Therapists who are modern day Elizabeth Cassons. The stories of these Elizabeth Cassons span traditional Occupational Therapy roles, entrepreneurship, education, and innovative settings, such as social farming, and include all sorts of different people, from different backgrounds across the globe, who have had different trajectories. Each of the stories is a story of passion and the power of occupation. We need these inspirational stories now more than ever.

The stories also resonate with my challenge to Occupational Therapists in the RCOT Elizabeth Casson Memorial Lecture 2024, namely "for us to have reach and influence, it means we all have a part to play in creating a social movement. Making the choice to act, or not, matters." I also observed that people choose not to act for all sorts of reasons such as a lack of confidence, not knowing where to start, feeling too inexperienced or feeling too experienced, or feeling like they are not a leader. If you experience one or more of these barriers, this book is an excellent place to start overcoming them. Martina has not just captured significant achievements within Occupational Therapy but the stories behind the headlines. This shows that many of these achievements have happened despite the Occupational Therapists involved experiencing similar barriers.

*RCOT is the Royal College of Occupational Therapists in the UK. It is a respected membership organisation which supports OTs with resources and guidance and promotes the skills and profession of Occupational Therapy.

Be challenged

The stories reveal that challenge is good for us, and we become better Occupational Therapists by embracing it. That said, being a little scared is a part of achieving goals. If you lack courage, you are not alone; the Occupational Therapists in these stories have felt similarly. Some, like Rachel Brimblecombe, describe becoming burnt out and at a crossroads before experiencing a turning point in their career. As well as lacking in confidence at the start of a new initiative, our confidence can be knocked along the way. Martina describes how she experienced setbacks but also how these setbacks kickstarted further developments in her business. Thus demonstrating, whilst we may need courage, we can make brave decisions. It also suggests letting a lack of confidence shape what we do is the issue, not having a lack of confidence. In Martina's words 'When your passion and purpose are greater than your fears and excuses, you will find a way.'

Be inspired

If you don't know where to start, be reassured, many of the interviewees 'found their passion' along the way. They did not necessarily start their careers with a burning passion. Sarah Solomon describes being caught by surprise by her interest in motor neurone disease. Kate Sheehan shares how she developed a passion for housing whilst working in social services: 'I suddenly realised regardless of what your impairment is or what disability you have, whether it's physical, mental health or cognitive, your home is key to everything!' Paraig O'Brien has been inspired at many different points in his career and made important contributions to practice, service development, policy, legislation and, in retirement, sailing for disabled people. Anna O'Loughlin has become an educator after 24 years in clinical practice. Collectively these stories show our only limitation is our imagination and that we can be inspired at any point in our careers.

Be an encourager

Martina and her interviewees all emphasised the support they have had along the way. Martina describes her 'encouragers' beautifully as people who give you courage. Julie Beck described how a senior Occupational Therapist just gave her confidence. Others mentioned lecturers who inspired them, support from family members, influential Occupational Therapy and multi-disciplinary team colleagues and supportive line managers. The stories demonstrate 'We all need an encourager.'

Read this book and then act

I urge you to read this book because it is an engaging read. Where else have you read about an Occupational Therapist being shot on a home visit? It has inspired me, and it will inspire you. It will affirm, or reignite, your passion for the power of occupation. When you have read the book—act—take the baton from Martina and release your inner Elizabeth Casson. Whether you need to find your own passion, or be an encourager of others, let's use this inspiration to work together to realise the massive possibilities of our chosen career. The time is now.

Preface

'Each and every one of us needs to find
our 'inner' Elizabeth Casson whether
it's adding new plot lines to our story or
telling our story.'

This was the call to action from Professor Katrina Bannigan at the end of the 2024 Elizabeth Casson Memorial lecture. Elizabeth Casson was the founder of Occupational Therapy in the UK, she set up the first school in Bristol and each year there is a lecture in her memory. As I listened to Professor Bannigan in April 2024, I was already halfway through writing this book to tell my story and other heartfelt stories of Occupational Therapists (OTs) from across the world who are making a huge difference to the people and communities they serve, as well as to their profession. I had already decided that as an Occupational Therapist of 40 years, I wanted to tell my story to inspire others about this special profession and to re-engage OTs who may be feeling less empowered and undervalued.

I qualified as an OT in 1983. For the first 18 years of my career, I was fortunate to have had the opportunity to work in a wide variety of settings all within the National Health Service (NHS)* in Northern Ireland. I gained experience in stroke rehabilitation in a hospital environment, I worked as a community OT involved

*A publicly funded healthcare system in the United Kingdom. It provides a wide range of medical services, including hospital care, general practice, and preventive services, primarily funded through taxation. The NHS aims to ensure that healthcare is accessible to all residents, free at the point of use, regardless of their financial situation.

in the provision of specialist equipment and adaptations and I also gained experience in community mental health. This gave me a solid foundation when I decided to go into private practice. In 2001, I set up the first privately run assessment centre in Northern Ireland supported by my husband, James and my family. Over the past twenty years the business has grown and is now run by my three sons, Jonathan, Ryan and Martin Tierney. My daughter Louise worked in the business while she was studying but decided to go in a different direction and now runs her own bridal businesses.

Since 2014 a recurring idea kept popping into my head of writing a book to record family memories and to leave a legacy for my children and grandchildren. The idea was sparked by reflection following the death of my husband and I was pleased to finally published the book 'The Stairway of My Life' nine years later in 2023.

Initially it was meant for family only, as I never considered that it would be of interest to anyone outside the family. I was wrong. Gradually people started hearing about the book and so I began to give out copies to those who showed an interest. Then I was urged to put it on Amazon to make it more widely available. I was overwhelmed by how my story resonated with so many people. Many shared with me how my early childhood days were like theirs and how the stories in the book brought back great memories for them. Others who knew me from school were eager to reminisce about the recollections of our school days. And then there were the Occupational Therapists. Many who contacted me told me they were inspired by my journey, encouraged by how I built a successful business based on Occupational Therapy values and were stimulated by how their profession had the potential to allow them to fulfil their dreams and goals.

Some OTs who contacted me confessed they had been ready to leave the profession until they heard my story, others were keen to start their own business and there were others again who just appreciated that OT had a great influence on my life and the life of my family. They wanted to know how they too could use the skills of their profession to have a greater impact. I found many of them had lost their spirit and energy for the profession due to pressures at work, lack of funding, not to mention the extreme pressure COVID-19 put on everyone.

I then realised that many Occupational Therapists did not fully recognise the massive possibilities of their chosen career and the impact it could have on patients, their families but also on themselves as individuals and their own families.

Occupational Therapy has everything you need in a career. It has the capacity to provide endless fulfilment in your job, financial independence for you and your family and it can be used as a vehicle to help you achieve any ambitions you may have harboured but which have yet to materialise. It has the power to completely change people's lives.

And so, I was stirred to write another book. This time aimed primarily at Occupational Therapists but it is also for any clinician who may feel disillusioned in their current practice, who may feel undervalued or deadlocked. I want to share with you how I found my worth in Occupational Therapy. How I went from a shy, insecure and hesitant Occupational Therapist to one who knows the true Power of OT.

I have been an OT now for four decades and I still hear OTs say that people don't understand what we do. But I once read a quote from an OT who said 'We are no longer a young profession, we are no longer adolescents, it's time we grew up...' (Unknown) So now I feel it's time to take that advice and grow up.

As an OT nearing the end of my formal working life, I have had time to consider and evaluate my own career and profession and I'm extremely proud of it. For over twenty years I have worked in the private sector but during that time I have been providing support, training, advice and help to colleagues working within the public sector.

It is my desire that current and future OTs appreciate their value and continue to realise that 'We are responsible for other people's lack of understanding of our profession, it is up to us to show and prove what OT is.' (Turner)

Introduction

This book is written in two parts. In the first part I will discuss my OT journey sharing case studies that have changed how I look at my life and my profession. I will also include uplifting stories on how patients' lives have been transformed through Occupational Therapy. I will talk about how I gradually moved from being an insecure OT who was uncertain about my choice of career, to one who is proud to be part of this remarkable profession. I will focus on the variety of options available to OTs throughout their career both in public and private sectors and how we can combine both for the benefit of the patient as well as the OT. You will discover the flexibility that an OT career can give you and the satisfaction you get from seeing a patient progress and regain independence and self-worth through Occupational Therapy intervention.

In the second part of the book I will share interviews with Occupational Therapists who have really found and unlocked the Power of OT. The contributors are from both public and private sectors or a combination of both, and all have left an indelible mark on the patients and families they have worked with, and they have now also left an indelible memory for me.

This book is guaranteed to inspire and reinvigorate Occupational Therapists in your everyday work or help you understand what the role really involves if you are considering it as a career. We have stories from California to the outback of Australia; from hippotherapy in Ireland to an automated chicken coop opener in England; from planting sunflowers in Stoke on Trent to cigarette lighter modifications in Melbourne. The book is as varied and interesting as Occupational Therapy is itself, and I hope reading it inspires you as much as writing it has inspired me.

Part I

My Story

"Occupational Therapy.
Hopeless into hope.
Can't into can.
Impossible into possible."

Valerie Peña

1

'Just' Basket Weavers

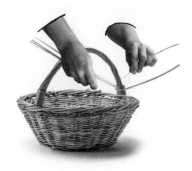

In 1980 I was studying for my 'A' Levels and considering my future career. At 18, I didn't have a clear plan, but I knew I had to decide soon as the university application form needed to be completed. I had three older sisters who were nurses. The caring profession appealed to me, but in the 1980s my sisters' stories of long hours on the wards, bed baths and bedpans as well as the strict matrons did not attract me. So, I studied the prospectus from the Polytechnic in Belfast (now Ulster University) to see if there was anything in the caring professions that would interest me. I didn't take physics at school as I didn't like it, so physiotherapy was out. I came across Occupational Therapy but had no idea what it was. I asked my sister and she said, 'Oh yes they have a cushy wee number,* they come on to the wards and help the patients get dressed.'

I thought, 'Well, I could do that but there must be more to it.' I made an appointment at the local hospital to visit the OT department and learned enough about it to capture my interest. I applied for the three-year course and for the acceptance interview I had to write an essay titled 'What is Occupational Therapy?'

---

* 'A cushy wee number' is a colloquial term meaning a job that is very easy, without too much effort or stress.

Because I had visited the hospital and talked to my sister, I had a one-dimensional view but it was enough to get me on to the course.

So, I entered the profession with a somewhat blinkered view and a very limited notion about what it actually entailed. But many times over the past 40 years I have been very grateful for having been guided to this profession. I now believe that I was always meant to be an OT. I have been able to use my skills to transform the lives of many people across the world. In the early days it was a challenge, but the struggles were most definitely worth it.

When I was asked 'What are you studying?' I always had to explain what OT was, no one ever knew. Even when we started going out on clinical placements, we were introducing ourselves and our profession to other members of the team. One of the first things we learned in our first week at college was a definition of OT so that we could explain it to others. At that time there was a stereotypical view that OTs were 'just' basket weavers, 'just' tea makers or 'just' equipment providers. From very early on I saw the huge potential within OT and I wanted to educate others. I had an awareness of the potential of OT, and I knew that the right OT with the right attitude could transform a person's life.

To move our profession forward we need to continuously improve by keeping up with ongoing research, continual education and embracing new opportunities.

I have had a wide and varied career which has challenged me, given me immense fulfilment and the opportunity to pursue personal ambitions but I don't believe that OT can honestly be described as 'a cushy wee number!'

Martina's Key Takeaway: OT is more of a vocation than a job, It's about finding your true calling and living a life that aligns with your values and passions. It's about doing work that brings you joy and fulfilment and using your unique talents to make a positive impact on the world.

2

The Surgeon

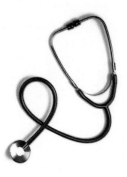

In 1983, I got my first job as a freshly qualified Basic Grade Occupational Therapist in my local community hospital. On the first day I was given a patient list - I was the only OT working with inpatients, responsible for the assessment and treatment of the stroke patients. Back then there was no induction, no training, you just got on with the job.

When I looked at this patient list on my first day my heart did a flip, and I could feel the butterflies churn in my stomach. I was too afraid to express my concern to my superior as I thought that would be perceived as incompetence. But the issue was that my first patient was well-known to me!

However, before I talk about him, I need to set the scene so you can appreciate the magnitude of this first meeting. I grew up in the 1970s & 1980s in a very rural part of Northern Ireland where the local hospital was central to the community. It was run mainly by doctors and in this case a very eminent surgeon who had gained the respect of everyone in the area. As a child growing up, Mr B. was a household name. He was always on the radio and in the local papers fundraising for the hospital and everyone held him in high esteem. His great work was regularly discussed in our home. I remember looking at photographs in the newspaper of Mr B. at a fundraising event standing with his tuxedo and a row of ladies in beautiful ball gowns which was a world apart from the life I was living at that time.

So, who do you think my first patient was? The eminent surgeon, Mr B! As I recall this first meeting many years later, I still get those butterflies. I proceeded to the wards in this old hospital and to a private room at the top of the wide, marble staircase. Mr B. had just suffered his third stroke. He had very limited mobility, his arm was non-functional, but his cognitive ability was intact. Remember; I was a very shy person lacking in confidence about myself and my career choice and now I was faced with this formidable personality! I also felt that back then OT was undervalued by other professionals. How was I going to impress this surgeon?

I went in. I introduced myself and he started to quiz me about Occupational Therapy because this was a new profession to him. He had retired 10 years earlier and there had never been an OT in his hospital during his working career. He asked me about myself. He asked me about the course. He asked what subjects I covered. Then he asked me 'What are you going to do for me?'

When I explained everything I was going to do, he wanted to take part. He was a doer, his independence meant everything to him. He wanted to get back on his feet. He wanted to regain the use of his arm. He wanted to be able to dress himself and play golf again. I took him to the OT department every day. We did a variety of upper limb activities, balance activities and sit to stand activities. At times I felt these were very menial for someone of his esteem, but he didn't think that. He was a willing participant in everything I suggested, and he loved Occupational Therapy. I wanted him to think highly of me and the profession I represented and he saw its true value.

He challenged me and I became a better OT because of it. I read. I researched. I referred to a placement I had done on stroke and read my notes every night so that I had a plan of action for the following day.

This was something that continued throughout my career. I feel that we leave university with a qualification but that is not enough to sustain us over the course of our career. We need to continually upskill ourselves and adapt to the needs of the patients and organisations we represent. I always wanted to give my best and if I felt I needed to learn more or research more then that's what I did, to improve myself and therefore the service I was providing.

Because of this experience, I was more at ease with other patients, my confidence started to grow as well as my belief in OT and the important part it played in the rehabilitation of stroke patients. I knew then that OT was valuable and that set me on a course to prove to others that I belonged to a worthwhile profession. Thanks to this experience, I developed a lifelong interest in stroke rehab. Even now when I visit healthcare facilities around the world, I often see chairs that I designed being widely used in stroke units and it always makes me smile thinking back to Mr B.

The following year, I moved from that community hospital to a slightly larger hospital 20 miles away in Coleraine which had a modern, dedicated stroke facility and I was presented with new challenges. In the smaller hospital I had carved out a niche for myself. I had grown in confidence with my treatments and my patients, but I was really working single-handedly. In the new facility it was a much more multidisciplinary approach. I was working alongside other professionals and again my confidence took a downturn. I felt the other professions got more recognition from the Consultants than I did and this bothered me greatly. I knew what I could offer stroke patients, but the Consultant had no previous experience working with an OT and tended to refer more to the physiotherapy team. So, like my previous experience I was determined to show them what OT could do.

I was fortunate to have had a very supportive and progressive manager, Mrs Anne Campbell, who was the first OT to be employed in this new stroke unit. She had limited experience with stroke rehabilitation having just returned from a career break after raising her children, but she had the ear of the management and could get things done.

In 1984, OTs were scarce and still relatively unheard of in many of the more rural hospitals and there was a huge shortage of qualified staff. She arranged for me to go to London to complete a weeklong course on the Bobath Concept* which was a relatively new approach to stroke rehabilitation. Very few OTs from Northern Ireland had completed this course at the time, so it was a huge opportunity for me.

This training gave me a major boost in confidence and elevated my professional reputation with the Consultant as he was very interested in the new treatment concept. Gradually at ward rounds I was asked my opinion on the progress of the patients, he referred to me when they were considering discharge, and my opinion was valued.

I'd like to end this chapter with John's story. John was one of the long-term patients in the rehabilitation unit. He was a 30-year-old man who was involved in a road traffic collision and had suffered a major head injury. The unit was designed for patients aged 65 years and older but since he had a young wife and family who could not travel 60 miles each way to Belfast for visits and there was no other facility in the area to accommodate his complex needs, he was placed as an inpatient in the unit.

He soon became our star patient. He had a very dense hemiplegia, communication difficulties and was totally dependent for all self-care activities. As a team we treated him as an inpatient for two to three hours each day for over six months - we had the luxury back then of keeping him as an inpatient. It was very intensive treatment, but he was very keen to get back to as close to full fitness as possible. He was very enthusiastic about his rehabilitation and in particular loved OT as he could see that becoming independent in self-care activities meant he could get home to his family. He also needed to feel useful again and he always expressed his gratitude for the help we gave him. He said OT gave him his dignity back. He learned to walk again, transfer independently and he regained some function of his arm. He eventually learned to dress himself, cook small meals, and go home to his wife and children. As the OT, I was heavily involved in his discharge and liaising with his family. We arranged

The Bobath Concept, also known as neurodevelopmental treatment, is a problem-solving approach used in the evaluation and treatment of individuals with movement, tone, and functional impairments due to a lesion of the central nervous system.

many home visits prior to discharge so his young children could become aware of their father's needs, his aspirations and his results really showcased the impact OT could have and transformed the Consultant's opinion of OT.

For many years after John's discharge, he kept in touch regularly and even visited me at The Disability Centre, the private assessment business that I set up 18 years' later, but I'll share more about that in later chapters.

My years in the stroke unit working closely with the physiotherapists and speech and language therapists, provided me with a solid foundation for the remainder of my career. John was a superb advocate for OT and someone who bolstered my belief that I had chosen the right profession and I could make a real difference in people's lives.

'The lesson I learned here was that if I want to be respected and valued then I must earn it. Since I belonged to a relatively new profession it was essential that I educated not only the patients but also other professionals on how I could become a vital part of the team and how my patients can benefit from the Power of OT.'

In today's world we still need to prove our worth, we should constantly strive to be at the top of our profession, providing evidence on the value that OT can bring to our patients and organisations. As a profession we are needed now more than ever to assist with early discharge, to keep clients in their own homes for as long as possible and to reduce the burden on our hospital and emergency services.

There is growing demand for our input in Dementia Care, Mental Health, Paediatrics and many, many more services.

Martina's Key Takeaway: If you want to be respected and you want your profession to be respected then you must earn that respect through clinical excellence and continuous learning.

3

A Leap of Faith

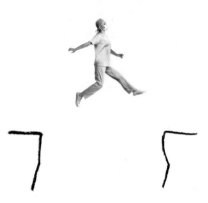

I have been very fortunate in life as I always had people who supported me and believed in me. I needed that support at various stages in my life as my self-confidence was low at times. Others often saw my value before I did. This is not unusual, I believe many of us do not know our true value and we constantly underestimate our own worth and capabilities. Even now I still need that reassurance that I am doing the right thing, and that I am still on track. I believe this is not a weakness so long you don't allow your apprehension and doubt to hold you back.

My first encourager was my mother, she raised a large family of thirteen, she was widowed when I was nine and my younger sister was six. But despite the large family and the enormous task of rearing a family single-handedly, she took an individual interest in each one of us. She never put pressure on us but when we aspired to achieve a particular goal, she was our greatest encourager.

My next great encourager was my husband James. It was clear from the start when I met him aged seventeen that I had met a true enthusiast. From the start he saw my value and believed in me when I didn't believe in myself. He never had any doubt that I would succeed, and he was the driving force behind my success. I was always drawn to the idea of running my own business as James had done this since he had left school. After working for over 18 years as an employee of the NHS, I decided I would like to start my own business. Previously I had been involved in many entrepreneurial ventures ranging from running a multi-level marketing business and a bed and breakfast guesthouse to being a style therapist and weight loss coach. However, while they were fun at the time, I didn't have a real passion for any of these adventures.

In 2000, I felt stifled in my job as an Occupational Therapist in the community due to major changes within the service and wanted to leave the job, but my other ventures were lacking in the fulfilment of helping people and not bringing in enough money yet. I was working part-time in the health service by this time, as I had a job share with another colleague called Joanne. We had worked together for years and shared some of my frustrations with work.

I heard a motivational speaker one time define an encourager as 'someone who gives you courage.' My encourager at that time came in the form of an OT. We all need an encourager in our lives. Joanne was that person for me.

'An encourager is someone who gives you courage.'

One day, she said, 'Martina, you know how you are always having business ideas? Why don't you set up a disabled living centre, like the one in Musgrave Hospital near Belfast?'

This was a place where people with disabilities could go and get a professional OT assessment for various pieces of equipment like wheelchairs, mobility scooters, specialised mattresses, reclining chairs, etc., before purchasing them. There was nothing like this in the northwest of Northern Ireland where I lived, so I immediately knew this could be a good idea.

As a professional group, we often talked about how a 'Disabled Living Centre' in our region would benefit the local community, but this fell on deaf ears and the Trust never did respond. Our clients who wanted to purchase equipment privately needed to travel two hours to Belfast for this service. Often, I visited clients who had purchased a wheelchair, a bed or a mobility scooter from salespeople without any advice or assessment and the equipment was simply not suitable. I saw that this was a service that was really needed.

After giving it some thought, I felt that this would be an exciting and worthy venture. Joanne said if I did it, she would leave her job as well, and we could do it together. This gave me the assurance I needed to make the leap of faith. Having the backing of another respected OT was what I needed to bolster my confidence. So, I went ahead and decided I was going to resign from my job.

James was working away from home at the time, I remember calling him to tell him I was leaving my job. He was very supportive, which encouraged me. He was not concerned about me leaving a 'good, secure, pensionable' job. He knew I had a drive to do something more and he was behind me all the way. I was willing to take a risk.

So, in September 2000 I started looking for suitable places to rent and found a very convenient new commercial unit in Greysteel, around seven miles from home. It was not very expensive either as it was part of a community project backed by European Union funding to revitalise the area, provide jobs and encourage innovation.

With the premises arranged, we contacted all the suppliers we had known through our Occupational Therapy work: suppliers of wheelchairs, beds, chairs, hoists, and so on. We explained we were Occupational Therapists setting up the centre as a private business and asked whether they would provide us with products to enable us to carry out assessments. We also asked for a discount in return for selling their products. If you don't ask, you don't get… Very soon the unit was filled with equipment the suppliers donated to us, including one supplier who even came and fitted a stairlift. It was very exciting to see it all come together.

At first, I didn't want clients to pay for assessments, so I got the money for client assessments from the suppliers instead. For example, they would sell me the chair for £600 and I charged the clients £700, which was the same retail price they would have paid if they bought the chair direct, but now they got a professional assessment and proper set-up to ensure the equipment met their needs. We also carried out follow-up visits once the equipment was installed. I didn't add on any money. I felt this was important from an ethical point of view. As an Occupational Therapist, I didn't want to make profits from patients. When one supplier heard this, he said I would only succeed in business if I lost my 'health service mentality.' But I never did! To me, health service mentality means putting the patient first. This is what I have done throughout my career and what has now become instilled in all the team at Seating Matters, the therapeutic chair business which grew from the beginnings in the Disability Centre. It's a clinical company where the needs of the patients always come first. We assess patients, see what they need, and then we provide the product to meet their needs. We will revisit the Seating Matters story in a later chapter.

Doing assessments in those early days I was occasionally challenged by other healthcare professionals who complained that I was 'making money' out of my patients. There were very few private OTs in N. Ireland at that time, the concept was new, but I had a vision and knew that we would be able to provide a valuable service. We were simply ensuring that the equipment already being purchased privately was actually going to meet the needs of the client. Until then, this often wasn't the case and many well-meaning families were wasting money on unsuitable products.

My job in the health service ended abruptly when one day, before Christmas 2000, I saw that the wishes of a client weren't being considered in the equipment plan being insisted upon by the health service. I felt that the decision makers were too far removed from the real-world needs of the clients and I wanted to leave my patients with a better personal experience. I left sooner than I had planned and I was nervous, but the time had come to make a fresh start. I was ready to take the next step and help more clients by going into business full-time.

Martina's Key Takeaway: For me, the key to my success was having an encourager at various times in my life. It is someone who gives you courage. Courage to take that first step, to follow your desires and to never give up. You never know how much a small encouragement can change the projection of another person's life.

"A goal should be something
that excites you a lot
and scares you a little."

Joe Vitale

4

Feel the Fear and do it Anyway

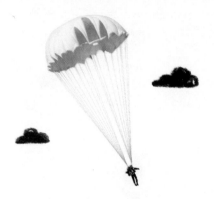

By March 2001 everything was in place, and we began building the business. We called it 'The Disability Centre.' Joanne and I agreed to job share like we had done in our health service job. I worked Monday, Tuesday and Wednesday, and Joanne worked Wednesday, Thursday and Friday – with Wednesday as our overlap day.

For the first few weeks I sat in the newly furnished, very quiet assessment room, ready to go, with all the equipment in place but there was no phone ringing, there were no customers knocking on the door and there were no buying orders. Those early days were quite frustrating because I couldn't leave in case somebody came in or telephoned. So, I was stuck there each week until Wednesday when Joanne came in. Then I could get out and start promoting the Occupational Therapy service. I went to nursing homes and other centres, promoting our work as much as I could.

On Thursdays and Fridays, my supposed days off, I kept promoting. I didn't go home and do whatever others do on days off – I knew I had to put the hours in to get the clients.

We had a busy open day and invited all local interested groups and individuals to view our equipment and learn about our services. We had media coverage from local newspapers and even got an interview on Channel 9, a local TV station at that time.

There was no social media to help us spread the word - it was very much a 'boots on the ground' approach.

The business started to grow, with clients asking for assessments in nursing homes and in their own homes. At this point, I decided we needed a van to transport the equipment. We bought a new Peugeot van which I was very proud of, even if it didn't have central locking!

Joanne is a very talented artist. Her passion was painting on her days off. So, she couldn't spend her days off promoting the business. I didn't mind – as I was happy to do it. I told her I was happy to continue if she was happy to cover the office for her three days as agreed.

While I was thriving on the chase and excitement of building the business, it was nerve-racking for Joanne. Around August 2002, she decided to return to work as an OT in the community. Joanne wanted certainty and security, which doesn't come easy when running your own business, especially in the early days. There were no guarantees, but I knew I wanted to make it work.

Joanne and I are still friends now, and while she has always been very supportive of the business, it just wasn't for her. Joanne had played her part in its success as her encouragement in the early days gave me the courage to pursue my ambitions.

Joanne returned to a job as a Senior OT and was very happy to split her week between her two passions – Occupational Therapy and painting. She never lost her enthusiasm for either and even in her retirement she volunteers at the local hospice doing craftwork with terminally ill patients. Once an OT, always an OT! You will hear more from Joanne later as she is one of the valuable contributors in the book. She will talk about her career after The Disability Centre and the particular interest she developed in motor neurone disease (MND.)

I persevered, determined to make the business work. I started doing medical legal assessments for solicitors to generate income until the business took off. This became a successful business which sustained me financially and it was important work for the individuals that I helped, but it was not what I wanted to do long-term. My sons were always enthusiastic from the start and very interested in the patients, the assessments and the equipment. I still remember them coming off the school bus and the first question they asked me was, 'Did you see any patients today, Mummy?' They were only at school, but they loved being part of the business and learning about how it all worked.

When I went into care homes to explain that we provided private assessments for equipment, care home staff showed me various issues they had with chairs. Elderly people were often sliding and falling from or slumped in their chairs. To me, this was not acceptable, especially as many of them spent long hours sitting each day. I came to realise that proper seating was a huge problem that needed to be addressed, especially for those who spent many hours sitting in a care facility or in their own home.

I upskilled myself with learning, research and practical training on seating and postural assessment. My awareness of seating and how it impacted the individual grew steadily. I knew that correct seating could have a lasting impact on patients and their caregivers, so I decided to concentrate on postural assessments and the provision of specialised seating. I had found my passion, and I was determined to learn as much as I could and share that knowledge with others.

Referrals began to increase as clinicians became more aware of the harmful effects of poor sitting on their patients and how proper seating not only helped the patient but reduced their workload as well. A company I was buying the chairs from was not keen on doing special adaptations for complex clients. It cost a lot of money and took weeks and weeks – a normal chair took four to six weeks, whereas a tailored chair could take up to twelve weeks. Following my assessment of the patient, I ordered in a standard chair and then asked my husband James to adapt it, whether it was the armrest raised up, the footrest changed, or the back adjusted. He adapted the chairs to suit whatever the patients needed. James was very skilled at this work - he had the technical ability, was creative, inventive, and always with the attitude, 'Everything is a challenge, nothing is a problem.' This is when James first had the idea, 'Why don't we just make our own chairs?'

It was a good idea but I had my clinical hat on and I was

concerned about the risks to patients should something go wrong, I was also uncertain about the financial investment. James tried to convince me that we could do it, saying if others could, we could too. It was food for thought, but I decided I wasn't ready yet.

After two years, we had outgrown our original location and we relocated the business to the large workshop beside our home. By this stage, I had built up a strong team with a receptionist, a couple of nurses to help with assessments, an Occupational Therapist I had previously worked with, and engineers to set up and repair chairs. I set up the new premises with James's help. Although he was never employed at The Disability Centre, he was always there to help and provide advice. It was a wise move. I had no rent to pay, and I was close to home, which proved to be crucial for everyone over the next few months as we continued to grow the business.

Martina's Key Takeaway: When your passion and purpose are greater than your fears and excuses, you will find a way.

5
Seating Matters

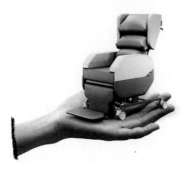

U p until 2008, we were still buying in chairs from a seating
company in the UK and adapting them to meet the specific
needs of the clients. I had become the main seating supplier of
therapeutic seating in Northern Ireland. In fact, most chairs being
used by the health service in Northern Ireland came from 'Martina
at The Disability Centre' which was how we were known then. It
was very rewarding to see the success of all the hard work. I had
gained a reputation of being the 'go-to' person for seating in N.
Ireland. But there were many challenges along the way.

The business continued to grow so I started to expand into
Dublin. There was another company in the south of Ireland which
was supplying the same products as me in the Dublin area. When
the other company found out we were in Dublin, they were not
happy for us to be operating on 'their patch.' I met with the man
running that business and explained that we were focusing more
on clinical solutions and told him that there was enough work
for everybody – it was a huge city, after all. I didn't think this
would be an issue, but looking back now I may have been thinking
more clinically than the importance of distributor relationships
and territories in a business. I continued working in Dublin. I
had written out a very clear goal in a diary which I actually still
have. I wanted us to be 'The Seating Supplier for Ireland.' A lofty

aspiration for someone whose initial plan was to serve just the local community, but I could see the impact I was having on patients and I wanted to spread the word. My purpose was becoming clearer every day.

We had been discussing going down the route of manufacturing and having our own brand of therapeutic chairs since James had first suggested it. While I had my reservations earlier, I eventually agreed to the idea. Initially, we were going to do it slowly because it was going to take time to get the designs right, secure the insurance, test the chairs, and so on. In the meantime, I decided The Disability Centre was going to get an injection of growth; I employed four new Seating Specialists from clinical backgrounds and trained them on our seating assessment process.

I wanted to ensure the quality of assessment was maintained. I was committed to providing a first-class clinical service to the patients. I had a plan in place for the areas we would cover. The more I worked, the more I realised how huge the need was and I had a sense of urgency to get it done.

Then, on 6 February 2008, I got a message saying the manufacturer who supplied our chairs wanted to meet. I thought that sounded very promising, perhaps they wanted to meet to find out about all our expansion plans and learn what I was planning for the year ahead.

The representative told me he and his colleague were flying into Belfast, and we agreed to meet at the airport. I will never forget that day. I was so excited and nervous to meet them. I made my way to the airport and sat down to wait. Then, a representative from the manufacturer came over to my table and handed an envelope to me. Upon opening the envelope, I was shocked to read the words: 'You are no longer a distributor of our product.' Our contract would be terminated at the end of March. It suddenly became apparent to me that the other supplier in the south, who was much more influential financially at that time, had put pressure on the manufacturers. I was beginning to see that for some, business came before the needs of the patient. I was doing a professional, clinical job, and I was enjoying seeing the difference I could make. I sat there with all my plans, devastated.

It was James's birthday, so we were booked to go out to a show although I was very upset. When we were out, James said to me, 'Never worry about it. We will just speed up the process of manufacturing our own chairs!'

I didn't see how it could be possible; we had so many orders and assessments already completed that would very likely convert into orders. How could we fulfil all those orders in time? It would take time to get our chairs to market even though we had, thankfully, already started the process. We calmly assessed what we had to do. I went through the completed assessments and buying orders. We ordered the chairs we needed to fulfil the current and any potential future orders, which was a big investment. We were taking a chance that the assessments carried out would all convert. Even our garage was full of chairs! I had enough to keep me going until our own products were ready to be launched. Then, a few days later I got a phone call from an Occupational Therapist who said, 'Martina, I don't know how to tell you this, but we are not able to purchase chairs from you anymore. The manufacturer has just sent out a letter to everybody in our organisation to say that you are no longer a supplier.' I was so confused. They had told me I still had until the end of March. Their letter to my customers also made it look as if I had done something wrong. It was incredibly stressful for me – not to mention I now had a workshop and garage full of chairs we had invested in with no way to sell them. Again, James was great, and his support was invaluable: his attitude was 'Keep your head down and get on with it.' Eventually the manufacturer sent a lorry to collect the chairs, however, my worries were not all gone. I had patients who needed chairs, they were already assessed, and I had promised a solution to their problem. I had these unfilled orders and more referrals coming in every day.

The period from March to May 2008 was very challenging from a business perspective - it seems like a blur now looking back. It was all systems go at the factory, by this time James and all three sons were working in the business. Martin ensured our chair designs were registered with our legal team and it was time to ramp up our manufacturing. We employed an upholsterer, sewers and a few other production workers, but otherwise we subcontracted most of the other work out to contacts James had for the woodwork, metal plates, welding, powder coating, etc. It was all done in haste, but we succeeded. Ryan had come to help with design and manufacturing and Jonathan was keeping the existing business going.

A funny story from this time was that Martin was still at school when we were designing the chairs but he had contacted a company who were the main suppliers of motors for specialised clinical beds and chairs across Europe and set up a meeting.

When Stephen from the company arrived at the office, he told the receptionist he was there for a 'meeting with Mr Martin Tierney.'

'He's not home from school yet,' she said.

When Martin hopped off the bus in his school uniform for the meeting, the representative couldn't believe it! To this day, each time I meet Stephen, he tells the story of Martin turning up to the first meeting with his school bag over his shoulder - he said he thought he was the victim of a prank!

Remarkably, we launched our chairs in June 2008 at a hotel in Belfast. We invited all the Occupational Therapists in Northern Ireland and the distributors who would potentially sell our chairs. I had developed a trusted relationship with the OTs and nursing home managers in N. Ireland and they were prepared to support me.

I always appreciated their loyalty; they saw me through a very difficult time and it's a loyalty that I now try to pay forward to our distributors and Seating Specialists. Today we only work with people who show respect to others, to me that is more valuable than money. I started this business as I saw a need to provide a service for the patient. That is the culture I have always tried to nurture in the family, and in everyone associated with Seating Matters. We brought on two distributors at the launch who are still working with us 16 years later.

'One measure of your success
will be the degree to which you
build up others who work with you.
While building up others, you will
build up yourself.'

Our accelerated growth caused a few teething problems and there were some issues with the chairs in the early days. We had, after all, been operating in a very pressured timeframe. Time was of the essence. Delay in getting our chairs out meant a delay in patient care and that our customers might source products from other suppliers so we needed to act fast. I discovered that my customers and clients didn't care about the teething problems, they just cared about how I dealt with them. They still tell us that everything was dealt with in the right way. If we had a small problem with a chair we fixed the problem or brought them a new chair, it was simple but effective customer support. Thankfully, although the manufacturing processes needed a little tweaking, the chair designs were safe and so I was reassured that patients were never at risk and no falls or injuries occurred.

After we began making our own chairs, we called ourselves Seating Matters at The Disability Centre. But that was a bit of a mouthful, so we cut it down to just Seating Matters. The name came about because I was passionate that seating really did matter to our patients and they have always been at the core of our business.

I debated whether or not to include this story but I think it illustrates that private practice and running your own business isn't all plain sailing. Sometimes the strain can really be a lot to handle. As a family we were always very aware of the need to keep a positive attitude especially when things were going against us, it helped us to find solutions to the various challenges which are inevitable in a phase of steep business growth. One such challenge was a legal follow-up from the manufacturers who had previously supplied me with chairs and a letter soon arrived saying they were taking us to court. The legal letters went back and forth for several months but I was certain that we had done nothing wrong. We could ill afford the cost of a lengthy legal battle and just wanted to get on with the creating clinical seating which I knew was so badly needed.

With all of this going on, we took a family holiday on a Bob Proctor* cruise. This was a motivational cruise with seminars delivered daily by renowned speakers. It was so good to get away together and get inspired, motivated and rejuvenated. When we were disembarking from the boat I was walking off the gang plank behind Martin when his phone bleeped. He answered it and with delight in his voice he announced, 'Mammy, they have decided to withdraw their case.'

A feeling of immense relief swept over me. It wasn't until that moment that I realised how much this had been dwelling on my mind. I felt euphoric, a weight had been lifted, and we were now ready to take on the world of seating.

Martina's Key Takeaway: Never give up. There are always tough times, regardless of what you do in life. You must be able to push through those times and maintain your focus.

Bob Proctor was a respected Canadian self-help author and lecturer whose teachings maintained the idea that positive thinking is critical for obtaining success.

6

The World Needs to Know

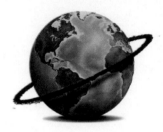

In 2009, my three sons were involved in the business in different ways and increasingly they shared my purpose and vision for Seating Matters. As a family it was all we talked about. When I had a remarkable outcome for a patient with one of our chairs, I enthusiastically told everyone about the difference we had made. The more complex the clients we helped, the greater our shared level of fulfilment. Ryan had made his mind up about the role he wanted to play in the business. His interest lay in manufacturing and setting up highly efficient processes to make the task of building high quality chairs easier.

Jonathan and Martin followed my training system and soon became experts at assessment and providing the right solution for each client. They had then, and continue to have now, a keen interest in the patient and their caregivers.

I believe that passion and belief are critical to the success of any venture or intervention. You must believe in what you are doing and in your own ability. You must have a real enthusiasm for whatever you do to make it work.

My purpose is to transfer the knowledge and passion I have for the necessity of seating assessment and provision of appropriate therapeutic chairs to clinicians across the world. I know that proper chairs are essential in reducing the risk of contractures and deformities, they reduce the risk of pressure injuries and the risk of falls, they help decrease agitation and promote comfort thereby increasing functional ability of the person. That's why I do what I do. That's my passion. What is yours? What will you do to make a difference? As Occupational Therapists you have the opportunity and the privilege to transform people's lives. But we need to really believe in ourselves and in our profession. Above all we need to have a passion for what we do.

Jonathan and Martin were determined to see if there were other OTs outside of Ireland who were having the same struggles with inappropriate seating as I had had before we made our own. One bank holiday weekend they announced out of the blue 'We're going to spread the word, we want to expand to England.'

We had relatives in the Northeast of England, so they decided to base themselves there to begin with. The week before leaving, Martin had set up meetings in Scotland with equipment providers and care homes. He would be travelling across Scotland anyway, so he wanted to make best use of his time.

Suddenly, they were heading away to promote the Seating Matters business. In Northern Ireland, people knew me and would happily try 'Martina's chairs' but in Scotland and England they were up against other well-established companies – including the manufacturer, who, until a few years before, was my main supplier. It was very difficult for them to begin with.

'I believe the passion we felt for our own brand of chairs and the belief we had in how they could make a difference not just to the patient but also the caregiver, contributed massively to our success.'

Nonetheless, they persevered by showing our chairs to as many potential clients as possible – in person. There was no email marketing, it was boots on the ground and relentless knocking on doors. They set up appointments, taking the chairs out to the patients and the customers. They often say that the quality and clinical benefits of the chairs often did the talking on their behalf. They set up 'Lunch and Learn' training events and I travelled over many times each month to help them deliver seminars and practical demonstrations of the importance of assessment and good seating. I provided clinical training to give as much credibility to Seating Matters as possible among clinicians. It took time to establish the brand and for people to trust a new company, but the business started to emerge and it really grew.

Jonathan, Ryan and Martin naturally fell into positions they felt comfortable with within Seating Matters:

Martin's strength is in clinical knowledge, business management and finance – he is very much the person to dot the i's and cross the t's; he is the driving force behind all our clinical research. His purpose is to provide the evidence necessary to allow us to transform healthcare globally. This will help us achieve our goal to make seating assessments and the provision of appropriate chairs a legal requirement.

Ryan's attention to detail and determination meant he was ideally suited to design and manufacturing. Gradually our chaotic manufacturing system was replaced with an efficient, 'lean'* system of continuous improvement all driven by Ryan. He researched how to manufacture efficiently and reduce waste. It was the start of a lean journey that has transformed our business and allowed us to create the best therapeutic seating available today for our patients.

Jonathan has always been a natural people person and thrives on meeting people and solving their problems, he has a passion for getting it right for the patient and giving the caregivers the means to care. He has gone from service expert and delivery

---

'Lean' thinking originated in Japanese manufacturing. The Seating Matters team have adopted their own 'lean' mindset throughout the business. This means having an intense focus on the customer, being hyper-vigilant about waste and always searching for ways to continuously improve in every activity whether it's welding steel or paying invoices.

driver at seventeen to leading a global team of distributors and Seating Specialists across the world. Currently, we have business throughout the UK and Ireland, Europe, Canada, USA, Australia and New Zealand with opportunities emerging in the Middle East and Asia.

I'm proud to say that we manufacture the best therapeutic seating in the world, and we are transforming the lives of thousands of people every year.

Today in 2024 there are sixty employees now at the Seating Matters factory in Northern Ireland with many more working remotely in different continents. Containers full of chairs leave every week for Australia, North America and Europe; and visitors from across the world come to tour our factory and to learn about our unique team culture and simple business efficiency. It's a world apart from where we started.

Seating Matters has become a success story across the world. I am amazed that the business has taken me to so many countries and there is no doubt that the decision I made twenty-three years ago to leave my job and follow my heart was the best decision I ever made. It has positively impacted my family and I would estimate more than a hundred thousand people globally. The success of the business can be contributed to my husband and family but also to the values of Occupational Therapy.

'My passion is to provide the patient and their family with the means to live a full and independent life for as long as possible and provide them with the equipment and comfort they need to maintain a good quality of life.
The Seating Matters purpose is to 'Give Caregivers the Means to Care."

I believe I was guided to be an Occupational Therapist even though in the early days I really was unaware of the impact I could have. I chose to take my career into the private sector as I felt I could have more control over my own day to day work and have a greater impact for my patients. Most OTs are contributing very positively to the lives of their patients whether it be in their health service, in public service or in private practice. I sincerely believe that the role of the OT in the community, hospital, prison etc., is vital and you can have a very fulfilled career supporting people in those environments. Sometimes we get overwhelmed by the magnitude of the task at hand and lose sight of the patient or family that is in front of us. We need to accept that we will never get it all done because things are always changing and in motion. I would like to share this story with you;

One day a man was walking along the beach when he noticed a boy picking something up and gently throwing it into the ocean. Approaching the boy, he asked, 'What are you doing?' The youth replied, 'Throwing starfish back into the ocean. The surf is up and the tide is going out. If I don't throw them back, they'll die.' 'Son,' the man said, 'don't you realise there are miles and miles of beach and hundreds of starfish? You can't make a difference!' After listening politely, the boy bent down, picked up another starfish, and threw it back into the surf. Then, smiling at the man, he said... 'I made a difference for that one.'

For those of you dedicated to OT, the "starfish story" is an important call to action, knowing that each life you touch matters, even if it is only one.

Martina's Key Takeaway: Success is not just about what you accomplish in life. It's about the lives you impact, how you treat others and what you inspire others to do. I want to inspire a new generation of OTs to have a passion and a purpose and to follow that passion for the benefit of others.

7

Change vs Transform Principle

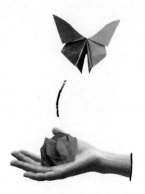

My passion and enthusiasm for OT has increased over the years as I see firsthand every day the difference I can make. For me Occupational Therapy is giving the person the tools and equipment they need to maintain or regain their independence thereby restoring their dignity, improving their quality of life and reducing risks to their health. At the same time, we are supporting the caregivers and the families by making their lives easier.

Recently I assessed a patient who had been in bed for one full year. Mary lives in a long-term care facility. She has advanced dementia and the care home found it difficult to seat her. She was sliding out of the standard chairs and was at high risk of falls, so she was put on bedrest. On initial assessment, Mary was in the foetal position, she suffered from paratonia and on first look she appeared to be in a very fixed posture. Her neck was flexed to the left side, both her arms were held tightly in flexion against her chest and her knees were flexed. She became very agitated and distressed when the carers tried to move her. I carried out an assessment and determined she had enough flexibility and movement to achieve a seated position. We transferred her out to the Seating Matters Phoenix chair using a full hoist and an in situ sling to reduce her transfers.

She was placed upright in the chair, she was able to move

her head to the right and look out the window, she did not have a fixed flexion deformity of her neck as was initially suspected. The chair was adjusted to meet her needs, she was given appropriate head support and after one hour she had both her arms placed comfortably on the armrest. Her feet were loaded on the footplate to provide sensory feedback on the soles of the feet.

I checked in a few days later and the nursing staff reported that Mary fed herself while sitting out – she hadn't been able to feed herself for a year! Other notable changes were a reduction in her agitation, more eye-to-eye contact and no slipping or sliding from the chair. The transformation in this lady was **remarkable** and the satisfaction I got from the outcome was immeasurable.

When I had first thought about what I would like to achieve in my work at Seating Matters I had a goal to be a major seating provider in Ireland. Then as we grew we expanded our vision to be 'Change the World of Healthcare Seating' and while this was an admirable goal, I ultimately realised that to 'change' was not enough. I needed to 'transform.'

So what is the difference between changing and transforming? To change something means to modify day-to-day actions to achieve desired results. But to transform something means to modify **core beliefs** and **long-term behaviours**, sometimes in profound ways, to achieve desired results. Therefore, to transform is much deeper, more long-term but ultimately more permanent.

No matter what you want to transform, you need to establish what those core beliefs and long-term behaviours are. You need to consider who holds these beliefs and how are you going to transform them. I will take the example of seating to demonstrate this principle.

What are the core beliefs most people hold about chairs?
Here are just a few:
- It's just a chair.
- A chair doesn't cause harm.
- A chair won't help to reduce one-to-one care.
- A chair will not help to reduce anxiety in patients with dementia and neurological conditions.
- The bed is more important than the chair.
- Seating and posture will not impact a person's functional ability.

What are some of the long-term behaviours associated with seating in healthcare?
- All chairs provided are the same size and shape regardless of the patient's postural needs.
- When someone has a pressure injury, they are put back on bedrest instead of sourcing a suitable chair.
- When someone has a pressure injury the first thought is that to upgrade the cushion for their chair without considering how the cushion is placed on the chair, may actually be the cause of the problem.

Who holds these beliefs?
- Purchasers
- Nurses
- Other medical staff
- Carers
- Family
- The person themselves

How do we transform their core beliefs and long-term behaviours?
- Providing proof by research and evidence.
- Education and training.
- Listening and responding.
- Real-life examples and other patient testimonials (at the end of the chapter I've included some examples of testimonials OTs who prescribed Seating Matters chairs.)

This is just one example, but you can apply the 'Change vs Transform Principle' to any situation you want to transform. I know I used it when I wanted to transform how other professionals viewed OT. I asked myself what are the core beliefs people have about OT? Who holds the beliefs and how can I transform them.

Each time I want to transform something I provide research, evidence, testimonials, education and training. I did this with my first patient, my second job in the stroke unit and again when I started working in the care homes. We continue to do this daily. It will never all be done, but we keep going because the result will be long-term and permanent.

If there's something you want to transform, this is a proven way to do it.

Testimonials provide evidence and a reference for others. Here are a few examples from Occupational Therapists who prescribed Seating Matters chairs as an intervention.

I provided a Seating Matters chair to a client with MND. Prior to OT involvement he had spent weeks unable to get out of bed due to not having a suitable chair. By providing a Seating Matters Sorrento he was able to engage with his family and environment again. He was much more comfortable and his quality of life improved massively. This is always a go-to chair for me.

Kirsten, Senior Occupational Therapist, Sydney, Australia

I had a young patient in their 20's who had acquired a brain injury with global weakness, no head control and no active range of movement. Following a thorough seating assessment, the patient was seated in a Seating Matters Phoenix chair which greatly improved interactions with family, staff and participation in Activities of Daily Living (ADLs) for therapy. It also reduced agitation greatly, provided sensory feedback and improved postural support.

Hiroshi, OT, Ontario, Canada

My client was discharged home from hospital with a suggested treatment plan of 'all care in bed.' She had increased tone particularly on her left side, upper and lower limb. She had poor sitting balance, was retropulsive in sitting,* and required assistance to remain upright. The client's husband felt it was important for his wife to get up, out of bed and into a chair. He felt strongly that a sense of normality was important for her. After the seating assessment was completed she was provided with a Seating Matters Sorrento chair. It meant we were able to introduce gradient sitting into the care plan instead of the suggested strategy of bed-based care. The client was able to sit out of bed for three hours at a time and appeared very happy and engaged. It meant a lot to her husband that she was able to spend time in other parts of the house and take part in activities such as family mealtimes. It was also noted that she had decreased chest infections due to less time spent in bed.

Alison, OT, Edinburgh, Scotland

Martina's Key Takeaway: Transformation is essential if you want to have a long-term impact. It takes time, courage and patience but it's worth the effort. What can you apply the 'Change vs Transform Principle' to?

* Retropulsion is a form of postural instability relating to balance and in sitting it means patients have a sensation of falling forwards or backwards when attempting to stand from a chair.

Part II

In Conversation With...

My primary reason for writing this book was to showcase Occupational Therapy and explore the diversity which exists within the profession. I want the public, other professionals, students, current and future OTs to have a comprehensive view of what Occupational Therapy is and how they can benefit from it.

To achieve this goal, I sat down with OTs from across the world who work in a wide variety of settings. The following interviews will demonstrate the impact they have had on their patients, their profession and how the profession has impacted their life.

The following chapters will take you on a journey which will enlighten, educate and entertain you.

Enjoy!

"Writing up a home visit on an elderly man and wanted to give a MASSIVE shout our to all the Occupational Therapists.

After his stroke they have transformed his life, they got him to climb the stairs, get in and out of the bath and got him cooking again. Amazing and underrated."

Dr Amir Khan GP

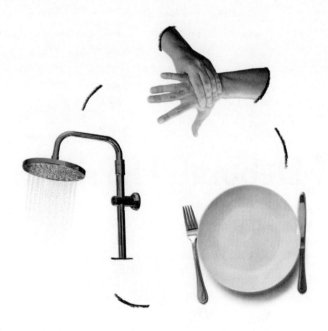

Why I Employ Occupational Therapists

Deborah Harrison

Nurse, Founder & Clinical Director
A1 Risk Solutions

UK

'For me, the Power of OT is in their ability to link different parts of an individual's life to form the best outcome for the person.'

D eborah Harrison is a nurse by profession who specialises in patient Moving and Handling. She realised the negative impact of poor handling techniques on both patient and caregiver and decided to set up a training course to improve outcomes for all.

Deborah and I have a lot of synergies in our approach to patient care and we share a vision to transform the way care is delivered. When an opportunity arose recently to combine forces, it seemed like a perfect meeting of minds and energies and we're both thrilled to have created a formal collaboration. We are both working towards the same goal of improving patient outcomes and giving the caregiver a means to care. Proper posture and an appropriate seating position can only be achieved if the Moving and Handling techniques are correct. Working together we will maximise the benefit to the patient.

Deborah began training others and eventually founded A1 Risk Solutions, a specialist Moving and Handling training organisation now accredited by the Royal Society for the Prevention of Accidents (RoSPA.) In her role as Clinical Director at A1 Risk Solutions, Deborah coordinates and delivers training across the UK alongside a team of OTs who are expert manual handling trainers.

In addition to employing Occupational Therapists she has also helped future OTs during her time working as an Honorary Lecturer in the Occupational Therapy Directorate at the University of Salford.

I invited Deborah to share a few thoughts for this book from the perspective of someone who, although she isn't an OT herself, is a huge Occupational Therapy champion.

Deborah, can you tell us why you choose to employ Occupational Therapists in your Moving and Handling training business and what you feel is the Power of OT?

Many of the trainers I employ to deliver training and services at A1 Risk Solutions are Occupational Therapists, and that's not by accident.

I believe that an Occupational Therapist makes an excellent trainer due to their client-centred mindset and open-minded approach to exploring solutions and overcoming challenges. They are big reflectors and therefore they can look at things from many different angles.

In Moving and Handling, the OT considers the individual's wishes and what they want out of life. A recent good example was a service user who sustained traumatic injuries after a car crash, who was experiencing pain on movement and was living an isolated existence in bed with infrequent visitors. The individual wished to visit family and friends or even meet them in a local community area.

Our Moving and Handling Specialist Occupational Therapist broke the tasks down into its key component parts, so it wasn't as daunting for the service user. They explored together how the individual could prepare to sit out in a chair for a long period, get washed, choose appropriate or adapted clothes, get dressed and have their hair done. They were able to assist carers with choosing comfortable slings as well as correct fitting and hoisting techniques. They also planned for how bathroom needs would be met when out in the community, considering the route and available facilities. The plan was a great success and the service user was eventually able to achieve their goal.

Our business largely involves delivering Moving and Handling training to healthcare professionals employed by NHS health trusts or local authorities for community care. Delegates are often Occupational Therapists and therefore having an OT as the trainer means they are well placed to engage delegates to explore the bigger picture and use their clinical reasoning to justify bespoke techniques and unique ways of working. This is so important as every individual has different challenges and the solution provided must be as unique as the client.

I'm honoured to contribute to a book about the Power of Occupational Therapy. I choose to surround myself with people from this amazing group and love working with them. For me, the Power of OT is in their ability to link different parts of an individual's life to form the best outcome for the person.

Martina's Key Takeaway: The natural skillset of an Occupational Therapist means they are a great member of any team, always keen to find a solution.

"Occupational Therapy
practitioners know that hope still
glimmers in the darkest hour."

Unknown

2

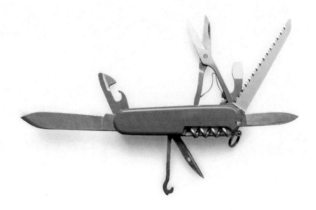

The Swiss Army Knife

Where there's a will, there's a way!

Maureen Clements

Community Occupational Therapist
Glasgow City Council

Scotland

'Passion is a powerful force
that drives us to pursue our dreams
and achieve greatness.
It ignites a fire within us, fuelling our
motivation and determination.'

Unknown

This is an exact description of Maureen. Maureen and I had one of the most inspiring and uplifting conversations about OT. If I wasn't an OT already, I would want to know more about it after having spoken with her! She made me proud to be in the profession and is someone who needs to get out and talk to students to inspire and motivate them.

Throughout 2024 I have met with Maureen several times as part of some research work we're undertaking alongside the Dementia Services Development Centre at the University of Stirling and local practitioners in Scotland. Her enthusiasm for care of the older person and her desire to transform how they are seated is fully aligned with my own goals.

Maureen had an inspirational story from the beginning of her OT journey and her passion for her profession and those she provides care for was evident throughout our conversation.

Maureen, can you tell us about your current role?

I'm currently working in a social services post as an Occupational Therapist in the community in Scotland. I work with children, adults and older people. It's a varied role which allows me to use skills I have gained throughout my career. I was drawn to the job for that reason, because historically I feel that Occupational Therapy within local authority was seen exclusively as equipment provision and adaptations. While this is still part of the job, the role has been further developed now to include many more aspects of mental health and rehabilitation. If we can rehabilitate someone then that would be part of our intervention. Most of the cases I have now are complex cases with people living with long-term conditions and disabilities but there is scope for rehab for some of these service users as well.

What did you do before becoming an OT?

I worked as a police officer. However, when our first son Craig was born, we didn't know at the time but later learned that he had some foetal distress at the time of the birth. Initially it was managed, but as he got older, we noticed he was not reaching his milestones. He was referred to speech and Language Therapy, Physiotherapy and occupational therapy, which we had never heard of. When we went along to the Royal Hospital for Sick Children in Glasgow that's when I first met an Occupational Therapist. She worked with Craig, assessed him and then told us unfortunately there was quite a waiting list for intervention.

I was really inspired by her to become an OT because I really liked her approach and what she was doing to try and help us as parents.

I became passionate about OT because I knew Craig needed it but the waiting time for him to be seen at that point was quite lengthy. I then thought as a parent I could help him if I could obtain the skills necessary. So, I decided that was what I was going to do. I also knew my job with the police wasn't going to suit because we had to spend a lot of time helping our son. I was working different shifts and there was unpredictability around my job. Whereas the Occupational Therapy job suited, and the hours were more manageable. So that's what inspired me.

So how did you make that transition from working as a police officer to becoming an OT student, it must have been difficult?

It was challenging in many ways, not least financially. I was working as a police officer which was well-paid, and going back to education again was daunting. I had only recently given birth to our second son Graham when I returned to education, he was eight weeks old, so it was challenging having to juggle being a parent, wife, working, studying and managing the day to day running of our house. I discussed everything with my husband, I felt so passionate about how I could help Craig and other children like him. So, my husband told me we will do whatever we have to do and make it work. So, I left the police force and went to work in a supermarket to get some extra money to help while I was studying. Sometimes I was doing a nightshift at a supermarket packing shelves and then going into university in the morning straight after my shift.

Was the university supportive?

Yes, they were fantastic. The university allowed me to record lectures on a Dictaphone because sometimes I was very tired from my many additional responsibilities. They were very understanding of the challenge of going back into education. There were times during the course that I thought 'Am I going to be able to do this, learn everything I need to know and get my degree?!'

Well, it's very interesting because there could be people reading this book that are in a career that's maybe not satisfying or fulfilling that would never, ever think of making that transition from their current job to OT. When you applied what were the personal skills you had that helped you get onto the course?

I first did an Access to Health studies course at a local college because the qualifications that I had from school were not relevant. I did have transferable skills from being a police officer, the ability to communicate with people, social and life skills etc. I was an older student but the good thing about that was for the first time I felt confident. If I didn't know something when I was younger at school and college, I wasn't able to put my hand up and say 'I'm not sure about that, could you explain that again?' Whereas being a bit older and having some life experience I was able to then say, 'Actually could you repeat that please?' There were definite positives about choosing that career a bit later in life.

Following completion of the access course I went to university and did a three-year OT course. I was committed to this at the time to assist my son and others who needed help. If I feel I can make a difference, then I will go off on a crusade! I thought if my son is affected by lengthy waiting times then there must be others who are affected too. They might need that help. I wasn't a qualified OT at that point, I was still learning, so I set up a local support group and my mum helped me out. We put out some flyers in the local community, some posters in the libraries etc. The Royal Hospital for Sick Children took some posters and they helped to promote it to other parents. The National Lottery gave us funding for some equipment that we could use so it was like a youth club for the children. We did lots of fun activities as well as looking at gross and fine motor skills in the background - it was fun! The parents were also able to support each other, they shared information about services, experiences and concerns. They were able to come and have a chat and a coffee and feel supported.

My mum and I used to load up a van on a Friday evening and drive down to the local church hall, the local authority gave it to us rent-free for a couple of hours every Friday for a few years. It's so lovely because the children from the group actually kept in contact which is very rewarding. They've gone on to various jobs – I believe one of them is working down in Wales with the health service.

I believe the paediatrician advised of things your son would never be able to do. Can you tell us a bit about his progress?

Yes, some of those things were very difficult to hear as a parent because Craig was our first child. We didn't know what our child should be doing at different stages, we had no manual! We were devastated, looking at this doctor with respect and thinking 'Well, she knows best.' She said his trunk control, his balance and his proprioception were so significantly impaired that it was reasonable to expect that he would not be able to do things like ride a bike.

But there's this part of me which is quite stubborn so I could not accept this and although he was delayed at becoming independent in riding his bike, we persevered with him, encouraged him to give it a go and keep trying. There's an old, disused railway line where we live, which has been made into a lovely footpath and that's where we took him to learn. We could see his balance wasn't so good initially, so we took him horse riding - he loves animals! While horse riding, we noticed he couldn't differentiate left and right so we painted the reins because he was good with colour - red for left, green for right. I hadn't considered hippotherapy up until that point, but being on the horse we were able to see his trunk control improving over time. He was getting stronger, and he was sitting more upright. Then after he had been doing that for a while, we put him back on the bike and he just took off. One day we were going along behind him, and he just started pedalling, he really loved his bike! A few years later we went to the Special Olympics, and he won three medals for cycling! This was the child we were told would probably never ride a bike, but I always told him;

'Don't ever let anyone tell you, you can't do something. Try many times, many times in different ways and then if you can't, then fine, you know you've tried.
Just don't let anyone tell you, you can't do something without first giving it a go.'

Craig is an adult now and living in his own tenancy. He is supported because there are some things that he still struggles with e.g., budgeting and organisation. However, he has gone on to drive his own car and he works in supported employment. This was a child we were told 'Don't have too many hopes for him.' He just keeps going on to achieve more and more.

This book is called 'The Power of Occupational Therapy,' but also in your story it's the power of the mother and the father. It's your power to give that encouragement, a never-give-up attitude. It's an attitude that fits in so well with Occupational Therapy to empower our patients to persevere and make the most of the skills they have and develop them further.

There's a desire and drive in me to inspire people to improve, particularly in situations of adversity, where they are facing significant challenges. The progress doesn't have to be groundbreaking, no matter how small the achievement is, it's worth celebrating. When my son achieved a goal, it may not have seemed huge to anyone else, but we thought it was marvellous. As parents we had the support of the whole community and a close family, and I think that support is important as OTs for us and for our patients. That's why I love being an OT. Yes, there are days where you're tired or there are different pressures and stresses, but I get my enthusiasm and fulfilment when someone says

'I wasn't able to do that before, but now I can because you have helped me or shown me a different way.'

That's what my job and my life is about. I always love when you can have a positive impact on someone, it's very powerful.

Apart from your son's story and the obvious impact you've had on him and the other children at that group, can you give me one or two examples where you felt that you had a positive impact on your patients?

I worked in a local care home where I had a dual role. I was the Deputy Manager but also the Occupational Therapist. I was the first OT to ever hold that position and I thought 'I'm going to do something a bit different here.' Many of the patients had mental health problems and advanced dementia.

Initially, I was faced with some challenges because some of the nursing staff said, 'Why have we got a Deputy who's an OT? It should be a nurse.' When I started working, I made it my focus to get to know the residents. I started to devise an activity plan for them as there wasn't a lot happening, they were sitting in their rooms or in the communal sitting areas watching TV with very little stimulation. I developed some group activities e.g., a walking group. We live in a lovely semi-rural village and there were residents who were mobile enough to go out and about. We started lunch clubs, keep fit groups, cinema days, quizzes, reminiscence, and music groups. It was challenging because some of the staff couldn't see the value in the groups I was doing. They were not invested, their attitude was 'What's the point?' They mistakenly held the opinion that the older people and residents were past a lot of these activities and unable to participate.

One resident stood out in my mind. She had advanced dementia, but we discovered she liked rock music. When the music was on, she would start clapping spontaneously along and vocalising, the staff had never seen or heard that before – they were not even aware she liked music. This was the beginning of the programme really gaining traction when the staff could see the benefit to the residents. While doing quizzes some people could remember interesting information and knowledge as their long-term memory was great. They were involved and could participate. There was huge value in that and over time the residents were waiting patiently for the activities and groups to begin each day.

I was nominated for a Scottish National Care Home award that year and won! I believe I won as this care home became a hub of activity, despite the challenges I faced at the beginning. It was determination and a belief in what I was doing for the benefit of the resident that kept me going. I just loved being able to look at a situation and say, 'How could that be improved? Can we do something better to improve someone's life?'

There's so much more to a person in a nursing home than just making sure they are fed and looked after. What about the other side of the person? What about the meaningful things that they could do? There's a lesson there for a lot of care homes to look more at Occupational Therapy because we look at things differently than the nursing staff do.

'Both my parents are retired nurses so I know just how valuable and important nursing is, but nurses and therapists often look at things differently.
OTs just have a different viewpoint. For example, we look at seating, how it can impact the person's function and quality of life within their environment.

We look at the whole person physically, emotionally and socially.'

I remember one gentleman who was placed in the wrong unit, and I realised his needs were not being met there. He was much more independent than the other residents so we got him transferred to a more appropriate unit where he could participate more fully.

It was quite challenging to go in as the only OT and be expected to deliver. I did have the support of the manager, and while I did feel the pressure, it was a great opportunity to showcase what Occupational Therapy can do. Getting recognised with the Care Home Award really made all the efforts worthwhile. I was very humbled because I was nominated by the families of the residents and other staff.

Where did this role fit into your career?

After I qualified, I worked in paediatrics for about 13 years - after all, that was my passion and reason for entering the profession in the first place. I did some sensory integration training and some other learning so that I could help our son. That was my specialism for those years, but I also knew I had an interest in working with older people that I wanted to pursue.

Older people really inspire me. They've often lived through war and great challenges; I think they should be given the opportunity to tell their stories and be listened to. That's one of the things I love about working with older people, it's not just about helping them or encouraging them to do things, it's also about listening to them, making them feel valued and learning from their experiences.

I created Life Story books for the residents in the care home. It was of huge benefit because other professionals or visitors who came in to see the resident could read their Life Story book. They used it to learn about that person's life, find out what and who was important to them, things they enjoyed. It could also be helpful if the resident became agitated or distressed, e.g., they could play the music they liked to reassure them or talk about their interests.

My daddy was diagnosed with dementia following my role in the care home and I did a Life Story book for him with his family tree and photographs in it, where he had lived as a child, his interests and likes/dislikes. It was beautiful for him to be able to look through it by himself or with family, carers and friends. It gave us all a talking point with Dad, and it meant he could recall some stories and events from his life that he could still remember and share them with us.

How would you like to see Occupational Therapy transformed in the future?

I would like to see more OTs based in primary care, in local doctor's offices and GP* surgeries where our patients can access us more readily. I think people (and that includes doctors) don't really understand what we do or the value that we can give.

If someone is coming in to see their doctor with early-stage dementia it would be very valuable to have an OT there at that point, to provide support or signpost to other services. At this stage we can maximise the person's independence as much as possible and support the family. We need to have a coordinated approach to dementia and other progressive conditions. One of the frustrations I had with my dad when he had dementia, was while there were so many people involved in his care no one was really taking the lead. Individually they were all doing fantastic work, but no one was pulling it all together. It's a frustration I had then and it's a passion of mine now to try and get this right. I loved working with older people and dementia, but I'm even more passionate about it now because it has impacted quite a few members of my family. We have a lot of teams in acute primary

*GP is short for General Practitioner and is a community based doctor with a wide range of general medical knowledge. They signpost or refer patients to specialist services when required.

care service, but services appear to be more reactive than proactive. We need to be getting involved with people and their families earlier in their journey.

Keeping people in their own home is less threatening and stressful that being admitted to hospital. Older people don't like going to hospital because it automatically implies that they are unwell. It would also reduce the pressure on hospital beds.

With early intervention that person with dementia might not feel quite so anxious because they're going to their local doctor which is a normal occurrence. It could mean they're having their needs met at the GP surgery or at home rather than having the anxiety and maybe trauma of being admitted to hospital where it can be a noisy and frightening environment with unfamiliar faces leading to further distress and confusion.

It would also reduce pressures on staff and the healthcare system benefits because actually we are potentially reducing those hospital admissions with earlier intervention.

'We need to be better at flying our flag.
Let the world know what we can do.
Occupational Therapy has a crucial role
in preventative medicine.

Keeping people out of hospital, keeping them
in the community, keeping them doing more
meaningful tasks that are beneficial to their
physical, emotional and mental health.'

What to you is the Power of OT?

We are so unique. We are so diverse as OTs, we're able to problem solve and be dynamic. We look at the person holistically, we enable people to live life as best they can, we try to motivate them to improve their quality of life, inspire them and encourage them to adapt to their changing circumstances. In Occupational Therapy there's never a dull moment, I'm constantly learning new things and learning from others.

The 'Swiss Army Knife' metaphor describes something or someone that is useful, multi-purposeful and adaptable. That's what I think of when I sum up the Power of OT.

Martina's Key Takeaway: When we actively listen to older people's stories, we validate their experiences and emotions. It fosters a sense of connection and empathy, reducing feelings of isolation.

3

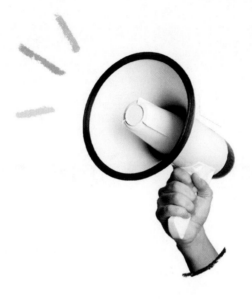

Giving the Patient a Voice

Kirsty O'Connor

Occupational Therapist & Clinical Training Manager
Seating Matters

Ireland

'I have a real passion for care of the older person and a particular interest in helping those living with dementia. I would love to see a transformation within the seating provision of care home facilities.'

In the last few years, I was looking for an OT to work at Seating Matters, to help represent me across the world and continue our clinical focus. I knew it had to be someone special. Someone who was passionate about seating and the impact it had on patients and someone who cared enough to always put the patient first. I needed someone who would help me achieve my goal of transforming healthcare seating and the clinical goals for Seating Matters.

Then I was introduced to Kirsty. Her personality, her passion and her personal journey immediately echoed everything I was looking for. I am proud to say she is now a member of the team and together we are transforming seating across the world.

What is your current role?

First and foremost I am an Occupational Therapist. I am now also the Clinical Training Manager at Seating Matters. This is a complex role with many different aspects to my job but everything I do is to promote and educate on the importance of seating and positioning for our clients.

My role involves seating assessments in the community and in people's own homes and hospitals. I host online webinars and face to face training events all over the world to promote and educate clinicians, care staff and families on the impact of poor posture and poor seating on patients who sit for long periods. I liaise with the design team at Seating Matters to provide clinical insights into product design and development. An important feature of my role is to conduct clinical research and clinical trials to provide an evidence base for therapeutic seating.

What sparked or initiated your interest in seeking this particular area of OT?

I was working for a private agency, mostly in long-term care homes working in care of the older person. The role involved a lot of seating assessments, but I really didn't feel confident as my undergraduate training didn't fully prepare me for the real world and care home environment I was working in. I hadn't had any seating training in my college years. I did a Bachelor of Science in mental health nursing, and I did a Master's in Occupational Therapy, but seating did not feature as an important topic on either course.

I was then working as an Occupational Therapist in the community dealing with long-term clients. I knew their poor posture and the inappropriate chairs they were using were exacerbating their healthcare problems. However, I felt I had a real lack of knowledge about seating, and I felt very under-skilled when it came to doing seating assessments. I decided that I needed to upskill in this area and develop my own competence and knowledge.

Then I came across the Seating Matters Online Academy, I went through each module one by one as well as reading the Clinician's Seating Handbook several times. This really helped me to improve my clinical understanding and increase my confidence when it came to seating assessments and chair provision.

I now know that seating impacts greatly on all patients and I am grateful for the opportunity to help spread the important message in my daily work.

Why did you become an OT in the first place, was there some one thing that led you into this profession?

When I was halfway through my degree in mental health nursing, I was involved in a very serious car accident which left me with a fractured C2 vertebrae at the top of my cervical spine and I also acquired a traumatic brain injury. After my injury I was in a coma for several weeks and when I regained consciousness, I was admitted to the National Rehabilitation Hospital in Dun Laoghaire, Co Dublin. At the time I didn't have any experience of Occupational Therapy or the role they had in rehabilitation. Even when I was working as a nurse I didn't have much of an understanding of the profession. However, when I was a patient myself, an OT who was a key member of my rehabilitation team opened my eyes to the profession. She really inspired me to pursue Occupational Therapy.

As a mental health nurse, I had heard of Occupational Therapy. I knew that OTs helped people with communication, social activities and activities of daily living. I also heard about OT within the paediatric setting treating those with autism and ADHD but I didn't really understand the profession as a whole or understand how varied the settings can be.

The OT that I met in the rehabilitation hospital really made an imprint in my mind. Of all the health professionals I met there she was the one who really listened to me and who asked me 'What do you want out of therapy?' She was genuinely interested in me and what I wanted. Other disciplines may have looked more on me as a patient, but she looked on me as a person, she really wanted to know what my personal goals were.

So, telling her my goals and saying them out loud made me believe that I could achieve them. That it could be possible for me to drive again, finish my nursing course and most importantly look after my two-year-old child. It gave me the determination I needed to work hard. These were my goals and with her help and encouragement I succeeded. I think as professionals, OTs are very holistic. It's not just about assessment or treatment, it's about the person. She really inspired me in my recovery and in pursuing my career in OT.

For years I searched for that OT, I wanted to say 'Thank you' and let her know the impact of that simple question she asked "What's important to you?' However, I couldn't remember her name or really anything other than she worked in that rehabilitation hospital at that time. It wasn't a lot to work with. Since I joined Seating Matters, and with telling my recovery journey more often it made me even more determined to find her.

The healthcare system across the world is changing so much. Where do you think as Occupational Therapists we can have the most impact?

I have a real passion for care of the older person and a particular interest in helping those living with dementia. I would love to see a transformation within the seating provision of care home facilities. I want to work towards mandatory, personalised seating assessments for people in long-term care. I believe that everyone deserves and has the right to proper equipment that meets their needs and in fact I read a study recently that stated 70% of residents in care homes have inappropriate seating.

There's a large proportion of people in residential care homes who have a diagnosis of dementia, and at Seating Matters we have enough evidence to prove that appropriate seating can have a profound impact on the lives of these clients. Dementia continues to be a growing problem and as OTs we can help to educate other clinicians, families and carers on the positive impact that proper assessment can have on quality of life. I see it every day and I feel compelled to spread the word.

At present there is a screening tool and risk assessment for pressure injury, falls and nutrition but there isn't one for seating. That's because there's such a lack of understanding of the importance of seating within all disciplines. We need a standardised screening tool that could be used within the multidisciplinary team (MDT) so nurses and other clinical staff can use it in long-term and acute care to help identify the risks associated with poor sitting in the wrong chair and to be able to recommend a seating assessment.

Can you tell me about one patient or scenario which proved the value you can give as an OT?

I can think of a patient straight away. I was asked to see a lady last year who had a diagnosis of dementia, and she was bedbound. The care staff weren't sure how to manage her. She presented with aggressive behaviours; she was falling from her bed regularly, so they used crash mats on the floor just to reduce risk of injury. When the staff attempted to seat her in a standard chair she became very distressed, partly due to very frequent use of hoists and partly due to discomfort and pain from a chair that didn't suit her body shape and size.

As a result, she remained on bedrest as she was not safe to sit out and the distress was too much for her and the staff. Following assessment and trial with an appropriate therapeutic chair the difference was dramatic and immediate. We hoisted her into the Seating Matters Atlanta chair and almost instantly as she touched the chair her muscle tone relaxed, her demeanour calmed, and she completely changed. She looked around the room and began engaging with people. Watching this scene was amazing, she began to interact with the fidget toy, and she reached for a biscuit which was on the table. She would never have done any of this when in bed. We left the chair for a couple of days until her own Seating Matters Atlanta chair was delivered. Staff reported that there were no more falls because they were able to transfer her easily onto the chair and bring her out to the day rooms to engage with other people. It really made such a difference to her life and the lives of her family because they could see the change too. The staff were very pleased as they reduced the requirement for one-to-one supervision and they had peace of mind that she was seated safely.

What do you think is the Power of OT?

I think that Occupational Therapy is so different to any other disciplines as we have always been trained to treat the person holistically. I spoke earlier about the OT I met when I was a patient in the rehab hospital. She was the one professional who made such an impact on me and made such a difference to my recovery simply by asking what I wanted. What was important to me? She simply gave me a say in my treatment plan. For me the Power of OT is giving our patients a voice.

Martina's Key Takeaway: Always consider the patients' goals and what is important to them. Sometimes we are so busy trying to do our job we forget to ask 'What matters to you?'

4

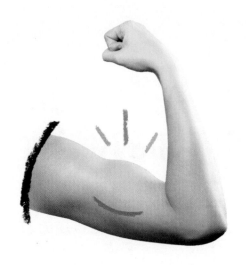

Restored Confidence
Through Intervention

Julie Beck

Community Senior Occupational Therapist
NHS

England

'It is about giving the person the confidence to use their skills. Often, they still have those skills, they just need the confidence in doing it again. I think as OTs we can project confidence onto the person and enable them through adaptation or rehabilitation to get their lives back again.'

I first met Julie when she made a visit to the Seating Matters factory in 2018. Her keen interest in therapeutic seating and the impact it could have with her patients led her to learn more about the assessment process, the provision of seating and the process of manufacturing. So, when I was looking for OTs for this book who went the extra mile for their patients, I knew I had to speak to Julie.

I interviewed her about her current role as an OT in reablement and her deep passion for her job was evident throughout the conversation. She has been an OT for many years, and I was so touched by the message in her follow up email that I thought I should include it:

'Getting the opportunity to be reflective about my career and my journey has absolutely energised me this morning. It's something we should all do every so often. I have always loved my profession and the power we give people to take back control of their lives enabling them to engage in occupations that are meaningful to them. In my 34th year as an OT I feel as enthusiastic now as I was then - who could ask for anything more?!'

Can you share an overview of your current role?

I work in a community-based role. It's a multidisciplinary team with Physiotherapists, Reablement Workers, Occupational Therapy Assistants (OTAs) and Technical Instructors (TIs). We run a six-week programme which is a short-term service to provide rehabilitation to patients either following a hospital discharge or for people who have long-term disabilities in the community.

For me, that is really the essence of Occupational Therapy, to provide this service in the patient's own home to promote independence and utilise their skills. We assess and advise not only on the self-care and functional skills, but it's also teaching them ways of using their leisure time and developing their interests.

Elizabeth Casson is widely recognised as the founder of Occupational Therapy in England and her philosophy championed the importance of meaningful occupation in rehabilitation and well-being.

I am currently working with a patient which exemplifies Elizabeth Casson's philosophy. The patient has always been very passionate about DIY and home improvements and is currently recovering following a stroke about eight months ago. We've been doing some grasp level one exercises with him to try and encourage that upper limb function again. Together with the patient we have decided that we're going to start using DIY as a way of encouraging these repetitive movements.

Why did you make the move into the reablement role?

After twenty-four years in a community post I was getting a little bit frustrated knowing that a client needed rehabilitation and more intervention than I could give in my role at that time. It was such a gap in service that it felt that you were just accommodating their disability as opposed to actively encouraging rehabilitation. My current role is very fulfilling, it's everything I hoped I would do as an OT when I first graduated from university. We are very successful in keeping people in the community, which reduces pressure on hospitals. I firmly believe it's a service which should be rolled out in more areas.

When I started my OT career, I was sponsored by a local authority for two years as they funded my OT course. So, when my course was complete, I went to work for the local authority. It was a baptism of fire going from being a university student to being the only OT in charge of and supervising support workers. I had to be so knowledgeable, it was scary and a huge learning curve. When we leave university, I don't think we are ready for the real-life work challenges. We learn on the job and continual postgraduate learning is vital to give the best service to our patients. To me, it's a lifelong learning curve in OT. If you get to a point where you feel like you have nothing left to learn, it could be time for personal and professional reflection.

Who is your inspiration or role model?

One of the most inspiring people for me was a senior OT in North Tyneside, Annie Errington. She has retired now, but she was so thorough and so knowledgeable she just gave me great confidence. When I thought 'I don't know what I'm doing,' she would sit down with me, and we talked. She never gave me the answer to the problem, but we discussed options and all relevant points to enable me to come to the solution myself. She was just fantastic.

Tell me about one of your greatest achievements.

It was some years ago when I was doing reablement in South Tyneside. This lady was referred to our service. She had COPD and was on a carousel of going into and out of hospital. She was highly anxious, terrified of being on her own and was at the point of saying 'I need to go into care, I can't keep doing this.'

At that time, we had a flat in the community where we could have a patient stay for a few weeks on an intensive rehabilitation programme. So, I devised a tailored plan for her. She attended an anxiety management group to learn relaxation techniques and ways to halt the anxiety before it became too much. We had a care team going in to help her with daily living tasks and personal care. When she was able to manage her anxieties, then I started a programme so that she could start to complete tasks herself independently. Although she was not able to live fully independently in the community, we did manage to get her into a supported living accommodation. This was a real success story as we were able to avoid placing her in a care home and demonstrated the power of treating the person as a whole and devising a personalised treatment plan.

This seems like a very intensive programme; did you go above and beyond for her or was this normal?

It is what I would always choose to do. I think because it was a brand-new service, nobody was telling me, 'You can't do that.' I think one of the frustrations with many OTs is the limited time that they get to spend with the patient. It is difficult for them to get involved in a fully holistic plan with a patient. It's also important to say that our multidisciplinary team works very well together. I've never come across this before in any previous job. Everyone's input is respected and valued equally, and the teamwork is invaluable to the patients' outcomes.

Where, in your opinion, can OTs add value in the future?

The key for me is that OT should be provided in the community as much as possible because prevention is better than treatment. It frees up the hospitals and GPs for the most vulnerable and sick who need urgent access to care.

OTs can help keep people in their own home, prolonging independence. Importantly, this also helps look after the wellbeing of the caregivers, giving the family or carers the support they need.

What do you think is the Power of OT?

It is about giving the person the confidence to use their skills. Often, they still have those skills, they just need the confidence in doing it again. I think as OTs we can project confidence onto the person and enable them through adaptation or rehabilitation to get their lives back again.

Just last year I had a patient who had had a serious fall. She had fractured her leg was very depressed and became very anxious. I was tasked with going in to treat her with a short, intensive six-week programme until her plaster came off. During this time, we discovered that the fall occurred when she slipped getting out of the shower cubicle. Since her fall she refused to go into that room never mind use the shower. She had a real fear. My goal was to increase her confidence so she would use the shower again. I eventually got her into the bathroom just by being calm and saying 'We can do this.' It took time and patience but that is what she needed.

When she finally stepped into the shower, she just broke down crying, she said 'I can't believe I've done it and that's down to you and your confidence in me.' I believe that's the Power of OT. To show them how to regain their lost skills and get their confidence back. Happily, she has not been back to our service and is managing very well in her own home since.

Martina's Key Takeaway: Independence means having autonomy over your own life. Being independent gives a person a strong sense of control – doing the things they want and need to do, when they want to do them.

"These collective journeys provide inspiration and pathways to creative careers that have future potential in the growth of the profession of Occupational Therapy.
It is recommended that each Occupational Therapist take the time to reflect on the 'why' that ignites your passion, your journey and how you can make a difference!"

Leeanne M. Carey, Sylvia Docker lecture

5

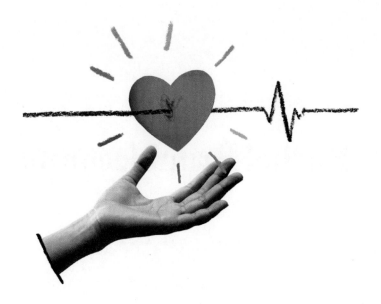

I Got My Heartbeat
Back Again

Rachel Brimblecombe

Occupational Therapist and Founder
Better Rehab

Sydney, Australia

'If as an OT, you get caught in an area
that is not 'filling your cup' anymore,
I would say instead of deciding
you no longer want to be an OT,
I believe it's important to think more
broadly and just try something else.'

Better Rehab is Australia's fastest-growing Allied Health provider, founded and run by Rachel Brimblecombe. I met Rachel in Melbourne when I was recently asked to present at the Better Rehab annual conference. Better Rehab was created to provide better support for people living with a disability, and to be a better place for therapists to work.

The therapists values guide their direction and decisions and they have helped make Better Rehab what it is today and will be in the future. Through in-home, in-clinic and telehealth services, their passionate, skilled clinicians help people aged 0-65 across Australia and New Zealand.

My admiration for what Rachel has achieved knows no bounds. She is a true advocate for Occupational Therapy and an inspiration to everyone.

So can you give me a brief outline of your current business and how it started?

Better Rehab started in my lounge room in 2017. I remember sitting there thinking 'I really want to make a difference,' but I didn't know what that looked like at the time. I had started my career as a Driving Assessment Occupational Therapist because that was my passion and I found it so rewarding. At that time, I was also lecturing to keep my skills current and one of the support coordinators from NDIS* said to me 'There's a great need for good OTs out there because it's just such an underutilised area. Would you be interested in doing Community Occupational Therapy?'

So that was how I transitioned into a Community OT role and honestly it just blew me away.

> **'As an OT we looked at the clients' goals that meant something to them, we looked at meaningful occupation and worked at getting our clients back to that.'**

I saw the potential and the impact I could have on the clients, then I began to think I can't do this by myself. I had a vision of putting people first and doing things a little bit differently. I was at that crossroads, so I decided if I was going to commit to the clients, I was going to do it well. That's when the growth started. I advertised for OTs. We just trained each other at the early stage, it's amazing seeing different perspectives and from there we just kept growing the OT division. The impetus to go into

The National Disability Insurance Scheme is how the Australian Government funds the costs associated with having a permanent and significant disability. This assists people with disability and their families to access the supports they need. The NDIS is overseen by the National Disability Insurance Agency (NDIA.)

other disciplines happened when I was looking for speech therapy services and I couldn't find any. When I did find therapists that specialised in high tech communications it was months or even years on a waiting list for my clients. I had really committed at this stage, and I wanted to be fully holistic in my approach. I needed to find the right people and train them up. That's how we started entering each discipline. As we came across barriers with other disciplines e.g., Physiotherapists and positive behaviour support workers, we decided to include them on the team so we could give the 360° support that the clients needed.

Tell me about how your OT career started?

My first role was in Queensland, and it was bit of a mishmash of different types of OT services. The experience helped me decide on the certain areas that I wasn't as passionate about, but I was thankful that it gave me a really rounded approach toward OT which I think is important early in an OT career. Then I went into the community setting and that was very specific. It was mostly about prescribing basic home modifications and wheelchairs, nothing complex at all. After that I went to a hospital with an exceptionally good neurological department which I loved. That's where I started developing a particular passion for neuro-care and I became a neuro-specialist. However, I kept reflecting on my first experience of the community setting which is interesting as I wasn't getting those outcomes that I really went into Occupational Therapy to achieve. While I had loved the hospital, I became burnt out and I was at a crossroads again where I didn't know what I wanted to do - I almost thought about giving up OT!

Then I was approached by a friend who told me about a position in this university, it was almost like a calling. It was a position as an OT lecturer specialising in neurology. So, I thought 'Why not?' I never expected to get it because I was only 24 at the time so I thought I was too young. I connected with the lecturers, and I honestly think it saved me.

'I went there, and I remembered why I did OT. The education, the support, training up the next generation, it all really reinvigorated me. It was like I got my heartbeat back again.'

Who was your role model or who inspired you?

I can tell you straight away that there is this amazing lecturer who really inspired me - she would be horrified if she knew I was speaking about her! She was Head of School then and has now progressed to an even higher position at ACU (Australian Catholic University.) She was an amazing leader, an amazing mentor, really inspiring in the way that she does things, very purposeful, very passionate about Occupational Therapy but all this in a very confident and inspiring way. She honestly is one of the reasons why I was really invigorated again because she was such a testament to how strong OTs can be. She trains in The CO-OP Approach* and has achieved a lot. It's so important to have that one person who keeps you going.

I am also very fortunate to have my executive team to support and inspire me. There are many in the team, but one in particular who complements the way that I think. I can talk to her, and she can process, reframe and deliver my ideas in such a special way that I wouldn't have thought of. My team are passionate about giving back and making a difference, if I'm ever feeling down all I need to do is give them a call and they will get me reenergised about what we're doing.

Cognitive Orientation to daily Occupational Performance (CO-OP Approach™) is a performance-based treatment approach for children and adults who experience difficulties performing the skills they want to, need to or are expected to. CO-OP is a tailored, client-centred approach involving collaborative goal setting, dynamic performance analysis, cognitive strategy use, guided discovery, and enabling principles.

Have you ever felt that OT could have been better acknowledged or accepted?

Absolutely! I went into OT just by chance, it wasn't intentional which is sad because it's such an amazing profession. I hadn't heard of OT specifically although I knew of Allied Health Professions (AHP) in general because I was born with a cleft pallet. I couldn't speak for several years, so I had to have corrective therapy for a very long time with intensive speech pathology. That fuelled my interest in AHP and when I was choosing a profession I stumbled across OT as I was looking at Speech Therapy. I remember thinking to myself 'Oh, this is more well-rounded and much better for me – it sounds almost too good to be true!'

At first, there wasn't that recognition, but since around 2021 in Australia there has been a complete shift because of NDIS. Unexpectedly, OTs have become one of the main areas of support and I think more schools in Australia are taking on an Occupational Therapist. What I've noticed is people finally know who we are and what we do. It's really lovely finally hearing people say 'Oh, I know someone who has had an OT.'

Clearly, starting a successful business is a major achievement, but is there any one personal interaction with a patient that you consider an achievement?

There are so many but there's one very important one. I had an interesting experience with a gentleman who was just a little bit older than me who was diagnosed with MND/ALS (Amyotrophic lateral sclerosis.) He was very angry about this because he saw himself as a real 'man's man' as an Aussie would say. He would claim 'I'd smash a six pack of beer in one sitting' and he swore like a pirate. It was a big identity crisis for him when he was diagnosed, he was so angry at the system, he was angry with everyone. He didn't want anyone to come in and see him. I went to see him at the hospital when I started Better Rehab. I walked in there and said 'Hi, how you going?' He just swore at me and tried to pick up a coffee cup and throw it in anger. I said, 'I'm just going to work with you, I need to prescribe a wheelchair.' He just kept swearing and eventually I said, 'You swear... I can swear too!'

I know that sounds awful but that was what I had to do to get him to listen. Then he said, 'OK love, go ahead.' and I measured him up for the wheelchair. He lived out in the Bush in Australia, so you can imagine we had to get him an all-terrain wheelchair to get around. That was how we started this very special relationship that lasted for the rest of his life. It wasn't very long, six months.

As he started declining, he started opening up to me about his family and his situation. At one time he was exploited by a carer and I helped him through that. When he passed away, he didn't have any family around because he had pushed them all away by that stage, so he tried to leave everything to me in his will! I did not take any of it of course but he wrote this really amazing note that was given to me when he passed away.

He said, 'You were one of the reasons why I could live in the last six months.' It was a really touching moment and very sad to see someone who was so formidable taken by such an awful disease. I think about that experience quite often, it was very emotional.

What's your ambition for the future in your company?

I've just seen the fundamental change we've made in Australia now happening in New Zealand where there is this huge energy and growth. I would love to take what we're doing even further in Australia and after that I would love to go to many other places in the world and impart that same energy. I'm hungry to make a difference in more countries than just the Pacific region.

Finally, what do you think is the Power of OT?

I think the Power of OT is the versatility and the fact that we partner with someone to develop goals that make a difference to them. At the end of the day when everything is said and done, we make a difference in their life and have a meaningful impact. We hold their hand until they feel strong enough to do it themselves.

If as an OT, you get caught in an area that is not 'filling your cup' anymore, I would say instead of deciding you no longer want to be an OT, I believe it's important to think more broadly and just try something else.

That is the benefit of what we do. We can affect change in so many different areas and I think that no other profession can do that, so I just say 'Hang in there and try something new.'

Martina's Key Takeaway: Never underestimate the valuable and important difference you can make for every patient or client you meet. The impact you make today can have a powerful effect on tomorrow.

"Occupational Therapists have so many opportunities for entrepreneurship because of the fundamental nature of their service: making a match between complex people and complex environments so that function and positive adaptation are maximized."

American Occupational Therapy Association (AOTA)

6

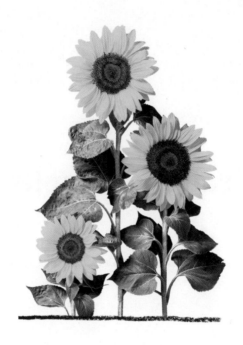

A Dying Wish

Karen Murphy

*Occupational Therapist, Certified Hand Therapist,
Owner & Director, Health Hub Professionals NI Ltd*

Northern Ireland

'I can't recommend it highly enough.
In Hand Therapy I have found my perfect
career within Occupational Therapy - I
can't think of any other job that
would suit me better.'

I first met Karen when I fractured my wrist in 2022. I was playing with my grandchildren and thought it would be a good idea to have a go on the hoverboard: It wasn't such a good idea! I had a nasty fall and needed surgery to stabilise the wrist. My daughter in law, Olivia, (who is also an OT and who we'll hear from later in this book,) had heard of Karen's reputation as an expert in upper limb rehabilitation and she recommended that I go to her for some additional rehab. I got an appointment as soon as possible after the surgery and Karen set me on the road to recovery. I had never been treated by an OT before and what struck me right away was not just her interest in the injury but it was as much about the emotional and psychological impact the injury had on me.

A wrist fracture might seem a simple injury, and in the larger scheme of disability, it is. But suddenly I could not drive, I could not look after my grandchildren, I couldn't do my hill walking, and the largest conference of the year was in England later that same week and I was due to present on both days!

In a few seconds my life changed, thankfully it was a temporary change, but Karen was very much aware of the impact and reassured me that my feelings of helplessness, fear, loss of confidence etc., were very normal. She just didn't treat me as a wrist injury, I was treated as a person. So, when I wanted to interview someone for this book it was natural that I wanted to include the only OT who had ever treated me. It was a pleasure to sit and talk with her.

Can you start by giving me an overview of your career and how it has progressed?

I am a Certified Hand Therapist, (CHT) which is actually a bit of a misnomer. Certified Hand Therapists are specialists in rehabilitation for the whole upper limb from your cervical spine to your fingertips, and we help all age ranges.

It's an American qualification and I became a certified in New York while I lived there. When I came home in 2009, it was to take the opportunity to set up the first hand therapy service within the NHS Western Trust in Northern Ireland under the auspices of two orthopaedic surgeons. When I took the post, I was the only hand therapist in the hospital covering a large geographical area, so I had to advocate for myself and my services to get the best for my clients. I didn't want to create a waiting list as the clients would become more chronically impaired; they would have more problems with getting back to doing the things that they love and enjoy, so I built a team. During those 11 years, I was limited in the referrals I could accept. I started to also provide my service at the local private hospital so I could offer care to people outside of what was available to them at the NHS hospital.

Then I decided to rent a room in an alternative therapies clinic in Derry and I was also doing medical legal work. By the time the pandemic came in 2020, I was working full-time in the Western Trust, I was working one or two evenings a week in the private hospital, and I was working two evenings and Saturdays in my clinic. I was very, very busy. I'm not sure how I did it; I'm not sure I could do it again! It came to the point where I needed a reduction of my hours, but that wasn't possible, so I bravely made the decision to work full-time in private practice. This allows me to use the full range of my skills as both an Occupational Therapist and a CHT. It's where I can give my best to the clients and see them not just as an upper limb or hand injury but as a whole person.

Certified Hand Therapy is a unique specialist area for OT, can you tell me more about it?

Certified hand therapists worldwide are about 80% Occupational Therapists and 20% Physiotherapists. The Hand Therapy Certification Commission has built a complete certification on upper limb rehabilitation.

The upper limb is a completely separate part of the anatomy, and in my experience, many Physios prefer not to work on the upper limb. As time has gone on and as rehabilitation has improved, research has continued to develop and surgical techniques have improved, making it a very specialist area for surgery and therapy. I've been studying it since 2004 and I am still learning - I don't think I will never know enough.

After an upper limb injury many people assume they need to go to physiotherapy which is fine of course but how do you think we can get OT / CHT to be considered at this early referral stage?

It's always a challenge to change people's perceptions but my best advocates are the people that I see, the people that I have worked with. When an OT becomes a Certified Hand Therapist, they learn the physio skills; the manipulation, the manual techniques, taping, exercise techniques, things like that. When a physiotherapist becomes a Certified Hand Therapist, they learn the splinting, activity analysis and a lot of the functional assessments. OTs are trained further in the functional aspects of rehabilitation.

We always say that we hand therapists are a special set, we don't really fit anywhere. We think differently. Physiotherapists who are hand therapists think differently to general physiotherapists and OTs who are hand therapists think differently to general OTs. I believe it's a niche specialism that you're either suited to or you're not.

For example, the exam that we take is extremely difficult. It is so specific and sensitive. It has been published that only 65% of people pass no matter how many times they take it! When you work through the British Association of Hand Therapy and become an Accredited Hand Therapist (AHT) which I also am, you can tailor your path to specialise in a certain area like Trauma and Orthopaedics, Rheumatology or Paediatrics.

Would you recommend therapists to enter this area of OT and would you ever consider training others to be Certified Hand Therapists?

I can't recommend it highly enough. In Hand Therapy I have found my perfect career within Occupational Therapy - I can't think of any other job that would suit me better. I now have a small community worldwide of wonderful connections through the power of social media and conferences. If I encounter a rehabilitation challenge that needs extra care or skill, I will tell the client. I will let them know that I know a therapist in another part of the world, and with their permission, I share the issue with them. I always find the answer. And that's what keeps me going.

Yes, I would love to train others however the main barrier at the moment is time. It's an incredibly complex course to learn and the student must be passionate and willing to do lots of work behind the scenes to become certified. I hope to be able to do this sometime in the future.

How important is it that you find a passion in OT, or in any job?

OT is so diverse, that's both a strength and a weakness. Yes, we can be anything that we want to be. But the challenge is that we are in danger of diluting the core skills and the tenets that Occupational Therapy is built on. So, if we can find our niche, we can find what makes us passionate, and use those skills to provide the best treatment and service to our clients so they are living their life to the full and doing what means most to them.

I think OTs often go into private practice because they find a niche that they are really passionate about, but which they feel unable to deliver upon fully when working in a public health system.

In our training, we are taught to be holistic: body, mind, and spirit. An OT told me once that when you go in to see a patient for the provision of a specific piece of equipment, it's difficult to be blinkered and just look at their needs for that one thing. We may see that the person has other needs but we are limited within the health service by time and resources to provide everything that the patient needs as quickly as we would like.

That was certainly the case for me. I had achieved so much in my 11 years in the NHS, but the day that I left was probably the hardest day of my life. I knew that I couldn't stay there and be the practitioner that I wanted to be.

What was one of your greatest achievements from a patient perspective?

I have so many of these, but I have a particular one that I always remember, and I wasn't even a hand therapist then! I was working in palliative care in Stoke on Trent in England. I had a patient who had 10 days left to live, and all this man could think of were his sunflowers in his greenhouse. Nobody was minding them and that's all that he could think of. So, I spoke to the physio who was working with me. The man had no relatives close by, so we got him out to repot two sunflowers from a greenhouse to a garden. That will forever be my lasting memory of him. He felt so much stress because nobody was taking care of them. To him it didn't matter if this was almost his last breath, he used it to do something he really wanted to do. Achieving this was the most important thing to him - he was totally transformed.

> 'Many of the patients I see feel powerless,
> they're in a service, they are the patient,
> they're with a clinician,
> but they are not in control.'

Another client who really stuck with me was a young 21-year-old man. I was working as a CHT in the NHS at the time. He was an apprentice with an electricity provider who had fallen and hung from a pole. He'd been caught by a safety harness but had injured his radial nerve, leaving him with a dropped wrist.

He was attending the Consultant who was mainly checking for nerve recovery. When this 21-year-old came to me he had grown a beard and wouldn't look at me in the eye. He couldn't do anything; he had lost his career; he had broken up with his girlfriend and was back in his mum's house. He had just lost everything and nothing seemed right. I educated him. I told him what was wrong in his wrist and why. I let him know what to expect as it was recovering and how long it would take. And he said, 'Nobody told me that, everybody was waiting, and I was waiting with everyone else, but we didn't know what to expect or how things were going to work out.'

The next time he was scheduled to see me he was shaven, looked me in the eye and spoke clearly. 'Right, what are we doing today?' It was tangible, he was empowered. His locus of control* changed to become internal. He started to believe he had control back, his thought process was 'I can do something about this, I am in control now.'

His wrist injury and his outlook started to improve. As he progressed, I helped him to become more functional and to continue to get better.' When he was discharged, he gave me a potted plant with a card. He wrote:

'You're the only one who believed that I had it in me to get better.'

Locus of control is the extent to which people believe that they, as opposed to external forces, have control over the outcome of events in their lives.

That has always stayed with me. This was a simple radial nerve damage, but to him it was everything. He thought his career, his life, his relationships were all over. I still see him out and about, he always stops to talk and it's lovely to hear about what's going on in his life.

What is the Power of OT?

The Power of OT is to make the intangible tangible. We came to OT with a functional brain to help people. We make things normal; we take things down to people's level; our power is in activity analysis and awareness of people and where they are at. We take time to sit down and listen to the person and educate them. If it's someone who is chronically ill, it may take a little more time, or a little more research, or a little more talking, but there's always an answer. That's what we're good at.

I think what happens to a lot of OTs is that they come to the point where they think their skills are just common sense... but they are most definitely not! Not everyone thinks as we do. We are carefully trained to think this way and we can forget this because it becomes part of us.

It makes all the difference to patients when they know there's somebody there to support them and help them understand what they're going through. I tell my patients, 'You're not on your own, we're a team now.'

Martina's Key Takeaway: As OTs we treat the whole person, not just the injury or the illness.

"Occupational Therapy practitioners help people live life to its fullest - no matter what. They provide practical solutions for success in everyday living and help people alter how they arrange their daily activities to maximize function, vitality, and productivity."

Florence Clark

7

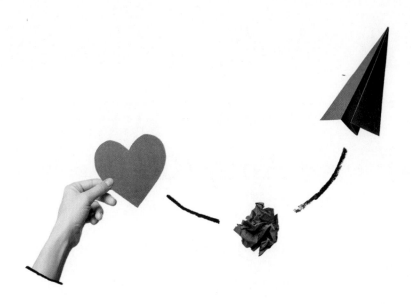

From Bedside to Boardroom

Andy Rich

Clinical Solutions Manager
Arjo Inc.

USA

'I think that's part of the key to the success of Occupational Therapy - our ability to bring function into what really motivates and empowers an individual.'

Andy Rich is an experienced Occupational Therapist who specialises in safe patient handling. He now provides excellent clinical guidance and support for all the team at Arjo Inc., a major healthcare equipment provider in the U.S. He is a renowned speaker at important clinical conferences and for our conversation I met him at the Seating Matters Head Office during a 2024 visit to Ireland.

We talked about how he has used his OT skills and creativity to help design safe patient handling products and programs that help both patients and caregivers to remain safe while receiving or providing care.

Andy received his Master of Science in Occupational Therapy at Rush University in Chicago, USA. Upon graduation in 1997, he worked in more traditional OT roles until he entered the world of safe patient handling in 2004. He has also served as a member of the board of directors for the U.S. Association of Safe Patient Handling Professionals.

It was a pleasure to sit with him and share his enthusiasm for OT.

How did you get into OT?

I didn't know anything about Occupational Therapy at high school. I went to college with the idea that was I wanted to be a Physical Therapist (PT) and after 10 credits of C in physics, it became clear that that option was not available to me! I got my bachelor's degree in Therapeutic Recreation, and I came out of school. I immediately started working in a post-acute transitional living centre in California helping those living with brain injury.

When they were stable and following the individual's hospital stay, they came to us. We worked in a Hacienda style house in the middle of a community - you wouldn't even have known it was a healthcare provider. We started working with people, getting them back to being able to dress themselves, feed themselves and to re-enter the community and the workplace. While doing that I started working very closely with Occupational Therapists and that's when I realised there was an exciting other career possibility out there for me.

So, once you decided upon Occupational Therapy, what did your early career involve?

Prior to 2004 I worked in a hospital on the rehabilitation unit and in ICU doing traditional Occupational Therapy interaction. Then I got injured during a transfer and needed to get off the unit for a couple of weeks, so I rotated to our Industrial Rehabilitation department. Here I provided therapy to facilitate the person's return to work. It just clicked. I loved that job. I really brought my OT skills into helping the facility create ways to allow people to do their job. One of our clients was a carpenter who was injured so we had him make small houses to re-skill him and give him the confidence to return to his job. I started developing ergonomic programs for safe patient handling and from there I became more aware of what was going on outside of the hospital environment. That's what led me down the path of bringing my skills to a commercial organisation in Arjo where I have been since.

Can you share an overview of your current role?

I am what's called a Clinical Solutions Manager for Arjo. While I'm not doing traditional Occupational Therapy in this role, I still carry those philosophies with me in everything I do. In my job, the main focus is to help healthcare providers work with individuals who have challenges in mobility. We bring in different types of devices - chairs, beds and lifts that all help healthcare providers be safe in moving patients but also help in facilitating the outcomes for those patients to get home, get back to what they were doing and to reduce any problems associated with falls and pressure injuries.

It's not a traditional OT role, but do you believe the skills you had as an OT coming into this role have influenced and helped with your work?

Absolutely! Having had the education and training of an Occupational Therapist, you just don't drop that mindset. It really drives everything that I've done, as we're looking at the importance of somebody's life choices, their roles and general occupations that can be affected by injury and disease.

Just recently we were talking with an individual of size. He was having discomfort when being assisted going to the bathroom. Everyone was acknowledging the importance of this man getting out of bed, but the other aspect is if this person is going to the bathroom, he needs to be able to do that comfortably and with dignity.

We need to make sure that what we are doing is meeting this person's needs in a dignified manner while keeping everyone safe - the patients, staff and other caregivers alike. Using my OT skills and training in my current job is vital to ensure the best outcomes for patient and carer.

Who has inspired you or been your role model?

My wife. Well, she wasn't my wife at the time, but she set my head straight and made me realise that I could do something meaningful with my life. She helped focus me and helped me get through school.

The next major influence was Polly Price Lackey, an OT who worked at the brain injury facility. She really helped me understand behavioural interventions and the importance of being a client advocate - all these important things that fall into the area of good Occupational Therapy. She really helped me grow up and realise this is something that I could do well.

How important is it to have mentor?

I do think it's important to have someone to check in with. To help guide you when you feel frustrated or stuck and to help you move forward. Having a mentor at different times in my career was very helpful for me.

Can you share any of your greatest achievements with patients?

I remember working with an individual that had multiple sclerosis (MS) and we were working on bathing and toilet transfers. We ended up using a patient lift called the SaraStedy which allowed us to help the lady get onto the toilet so she could go normally. As an OT we do so much work with activities of daily living - I sometimes joke that 'OTs kind of own the toilet!'

She said it was the first time she was able to go to the bathroom again on a toilet as opposed to having to use a bed pan. It was so important to her to be able to do it like she did before the disease started to take away her independence. It may seem like a very small thing, but it had a major impact on her self-esteem and maintained her dignity. We should never take for granted the small things that matter to our clients.

I think there's a tendency in healthcare for people to be very reductionistic and laser-focused on what we need to do. If a client has a head or spinal cord injury, the healthcare team can get so focused on the biomechanics of the movement, but through Occupational Therapy we tend to be more process-oriented and we look at the whole picture.

The individual who needs to be able to get up and go 'nose over toes' to stand, what does that really mean? The OT thinks this person needs to get up correctly to be able to vacuum or they need to be able to care for their mother or their daughter. It's about getting them back to what they did before. It's great that you can get up, but it's more important that as a parent you can bend over the crib and pick your baby up again without feeling the pain. It's through the techniques that the OT uses, how we look at the process and make changes that we really have the biggest impact on that individual's life.

In your business where do you see OT having the biggest impact?

Often what happens in business when we're dealing with healthcare providers is that they think very tactically, 'What am I going to do right now to take care of this specific task?' Whereas, I think OTs can really have a huge effect in how businesses and organisations are run through our ability to see the big picture. By looking at processes and systems we're able to really influence a broader way of thinking and ask strategic questions:

'For me to do what needs done for this patient, what are the systems that need to be in place?';

'What are the long-term goals for the person and organisation?';

'How does this activity really connect strategically with the organisation's overall goals?'

'With the way that we are trained and the way that we think, OTs fit in well, not just at the bedside but all the way up to the boardroom.'

Does your company employ many OTs and why?

Yes, we have a lot of Occupational Therapists working within the company. From a clinical standpoint they do a really good job and in addition when we are providing a product for a facility to assist with someone's mobility, the OT has credibility as someone who understands the individual's mobility and other needs. They can explain clinically why the intervention is needed and how it will benefit both the individual and the organisation. The are not salespeople, they advise clinically and with integrity. They can demonstrate how this will serve operationally and how the results fit with the strategic goals of the facility. OTs fit this role very well.

What do you believe is the Power of Occupational Therapy?

When you are working with an OT, our focus is on what matters to the individual. When we can find out what's important, we can use that to drive and design whatever type of therapeutic process we're going to intervene with. If I'm working with an individual who has had a total hip replacement I could work on range of movement but better yet, if I know that this person is a mechanic or a cook I can now create a way for this person to work on hip movement goals but in a very functional manner which becomes much more motivating for that individual. If I'm working with kids, another healthcare worker could have the child go through 25 repetitions of an activity it will probably not enjoy and have limited success. However, if we consider that the occupation of a child is to play, I can pull the 25 repetitions into a game the child likes to play and focus on the activity, I will get a much better response.

I remember working with a child who had 70% burns on her. We were working on developing her range of motion and balance. We created a gigantic board game, together. We made a giant dice out of a cardboard box, coloured it and painted it, all the while she was using all the required motions without even realising. Then we worked on throwing it and rolling it and suddenly she is completing all these therapeutic activities without even knowing it!

I think that's part of the key to the success of Occupational Therapy - our ability to bring function into what really motivates and empowers an individual.

Martina's Key Takeaway: Never underestimate your ability and the skills you have gained as an OT. Your skills can open many new opportunities and provide you with a varied and interesting career. You just need to believe in your own ability. It's never too late to start something new.

"Occupational Therapy is where science,
creativity and compassion collide."

Jessica Kensky

8

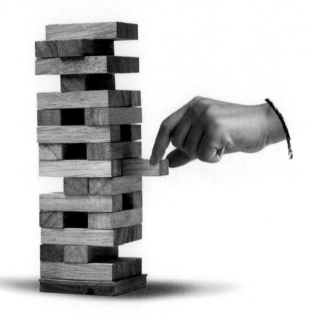

The Dignity of Risk

Sarah Solomon

Occupational Therapist
Committee Member, International Allied Professionals Forum

Melbourne, Australia

'Are you providing the input that you would like for someone you love?'

I was introduced to Sarah in Melbourne, Australia in 2023 while I was attending a conference there. She is recognised internationally as an expert and an advocate for clients with neurological conditions, but her particular interest is in MND. She is part of the International Allied Professionals Forum (IAPF) programme committee.

In December 2021, Sarah Solomon jointly won the International Alliance of ALS/MND Associations' Allied Health Professionals Award. When the award winner was announced, Jo Whitehouse from MND Victoria said;

'Ms. Solomon is known for her ability to think outside of the box to come up with a solution that meets the needs of the person with ALS/MND who she is working with or consulting about. She is a thought leader in the area of adjusting and adapting to rapidly changing function, and an expert on the assessment for and prescription of electronic assistive technology. She is a very worthy winner of this award.'

Sarah is also a fundraiser for a cause which is close to her heart, and in August 2022, she challenged herself to trek the Larapinta Trail in support of MND Victoria.

It was an honour to speak to her and share her thoughts in this book.

I'm delighted to have the opportunity to speak to you. I know that your contribution will be invaluable. Can we start by asking why OT?

I grew up in a rural community in Western Australia. My mum had some chronic health problems, and she was quite disabled throughout my childhood. We had a level-access shower installed in our house in 1978, which was the leakiest thing in the world – it was terrible! My mum was a nurse, her best friend was a physio, and she always had OTs in to help her.

I really had a sense that I wanted to work in a helping profession right from the beginning. It was always going to be OT, Physio or Speech Pathology for me... medicine came up a few times, but I thought I'd make a terrible doctor, so I parked that idea!

In the 1990s I did a school placement with a physio which, looking back probably wasn't the right kind of placement for me. It was orthopaedic patients in and out, and I just thought, 'Oh, I really don't want to do this.' I then started talking to my mum's OT and as I was a little bit alternative, it just seemed like the kind of job that would really suit me. That idea that the whole person was at the centre, it wasn't just looking at a sore knee or specific part of the body, it was looking at the person's overall needs which appealed to me. I applied directly into a tiny little Occupational Therapy school (only 40 students) based on campus at the rehab hospital in Perth. I wasn't the most organised student, but I had a lot of enthusiasm. My four best friends today are same girls that I met there.

I did my first OT job in Perth in a very small community, where there was a lot of support, and we had good supervision. I then went overseas to work in London. I did a rotation post and again I was fortunate to have had very good support and supervision. However, in saying that I'm the kind of person that if I don't know something, I'll go find it out. I'm not a sit back and wait for someone to tell me person, I'll push through.

I learned a lot at that time, from what I now know to be called 'reflective practice.' I remember doing things in my first couple of years where I didn't know what I was doing. I would think, 'Well

I won't do that again,' or 'I will do that a bit differently next time.' I think we can all learn a lot by doing and then reflecting on what you achieved or didn't achieve.

I believe that lifelong learning is so important for OTs to advance in their careers - would you agree?

I agree 100%. Every now and then it worries me that I've been at the MND clinic for 15 or 16 years. I always say to my junior staff, 'If I ever turn into that person that's just doing the same old thing and not growing and changing or still pushing and learning, then you need to tell me because it's time for me to retire!'

That is never the therapist I want to be. I want to stay ahead of the game, I want to make sure that I'm giving the best service that I can. If I don't know, I'll go find out. Things like reflective practice, lifelong learning, keeping links with colleagues, informal mentoring and peer support are imperative to allow us to keep doing a good job.

Can you give me an overview of your current role?

Since 2007, I have been working in Melbourne, Australia at the statewide progressive neurological diseases service at a hospital called Calvary Healthcare Bethlehem. We are the statewide service for people with progressive conditions. But the neurologists that I work with have a very predominant interest in helping people with motor neurone disease and Huntington's disease, as well as many of the other rarer progressive neuro syndromes. It is an adult-only service with inpatient and outpatient services, as well as a community palliative care service. We have an NDIS-funded service, and an over-65s service in the community. It has really grown in the time that I've been there.

How many Occupational Therapists do you have working with you?

We have 15 altogether across the services with a range of experiences. I'm the senior clinician in the neurology stream, then we have a senior clinician in the palliative care stream, and another in our NDIS service. The grading in Australia is a little bit different. We have senior clinicians which is a grade three, then grade two is the middle career therapists and grade ones are early career or new graduate therapists. When the junior staff start there is the ability to rotate through some of the different services to help with their learning.

To an Occupational Therapist reading this with no experience of MND, what is the impact that an OT can have?

When someone is faced with a sporadic, life-limiting condition, and their life has completely been turned on its head from what they thought might happen, the OT input (and I hope that I always do this,) is to give them hope. I give them hope that no matter the changes that are happening in their body, that they are still able to do the things that are important to them.

I think our real client-centredness, and understanding of the person and their environment and what is important to them is the magic of OT. There's no clinical pathway to how we can assist people. There's no magic set of rules, it's just around building rapport. People arrive worried when they come into clinic for the first time, often very recently after being diagnosed and there's a lot going on in their head. I'll say to them:

'Look, I'm here for the long run. We don't have a crystal ball, we're going to plan for the worst, but we're going to hope for the best and whatever is important to you, I will ensure that to the best of my ability and your ability that you can still do the things that are important to you.'

I talk about 'dancing the dance' a little bit with people with motor neurone disease. Often when people come into the clinic they have gone on Google and researched it, they have seen each of the stages and they just want to know everything. Our department is set like an independent living centre for people with motor neurone disease. We've got everything set up for demonstrations which sometimes leads the conversations or interactions that we're having with people. We don't go through a set series of questions, it's more of a dialogue.

I talk a lot about *dignity of risk*, about choices and giving them options. We talk about the pros and the cons, the risks and the benefits to everything. I stress that my job is not to tell the person what to do, it's to give them information to make choices on doing the things that are important to them.

I spoke at the International Conference of MND/ALS last year in Europe, on the dignity of risk, and enabling doing for people with motor neurone disease. I have seen a tendency over the last 15 years in therapists to be a little bit risk averse and it's something I would like to see less of.

I gave the example of a gentleman who had respiratory failure and no hand function. He was grieving terribly for what he had lost and was losing.

I simply sat down with him and asked, 'What do you want to do to improve the quality of your life?' and he said, 'I don't want to have to ask someone to light and hold my cigarettes and wipe my butt.'

We agreed then and there that that was what we were going to work on first. And we did. It created a sense that he felt I was listening to him and that I was engaged in things that were important to him. I knew that he also needed a bed, and we needed to look at his bathroom, but at that time those things were just not important to him, and I was never going to get any engagement. And so, by building trust, rapport and that client-centred mindset, we got him to be able to smoke by himself with a switch-adapted electric art lighter and a holder for it. Then we got him a bidet with foot control. They weren't huge, but they were very meaningful things for a man who was losing a lot of what was important to him. We regained something.

Was there anything that particularly triggered your interest in MND or did you just move into it organically?

My career has been really varied. I've just hit 29 years of being an OT and for the first 15 years I was overseas, predominantly working with young adults in the neurological rehab space. These were people who had had brain injuries, or a cerebral vascular accident and I sat well in that space. I worked at a Friedrichs ataxia* clinic and a movement disorders clinic, developing skills within the progressive neuro space. Then I had a baby and after maternity leave, I applied for a part-time job in a MND clinic. I had never really worked with people with MND, except for a short stint in the 1990s at King's College Hospital, London but things had been very different back then. It was interesting because I do remember feeling a little bit taken aback by the speed of progression. In people with Friedrichs ataxia, MS or Parkinson's, the progression is different, it's slower, longer.

So, I felt I needed to learn and read more about motor neurone disease. The more I worked with these clients, the more I thought 'This is the most fulfilling job that I've ever had in my life.' It caught me by surprise. Then it just started snowballing.

From there, I started developing more interest in it and I

Friedrichs ataxia is a rare, inherited progressive neurological condition.

stayed there. My first job was a year-long locum post covering someone else's maternity leave. Then they asked me to stay, and I got promoted - it was the right kind of space for me. Working with people with life-limiting conditions is not for everyone as things happen very quickly. It takes a certain type of personality to be able to cope with it.

Do you think you find it so fulfilling because there is a real urgency with these patients?

Yes, to get in and find out quickly what is important to the person and make it happen is very fulfilling. There is so much sadness that comes with the diagnosis - there's no cure and the doctors are saying, 'We can't give you a magic pill to make this go away.' But to me it feels like a real privilege to be involved with people at this very vulnerable time of their lives and to give that feeling of hope.

I am now very aware of the language I use. Slightly modifying the names of things or changing how I phrase things when talking to clients means that when they come to OT, we are changing the narrative of their diagnosis.

Rather than, 'There is no solution for this,' we say, 'What do you want to achieve?' and 'Let's work with what you can do.'

Another example is that I stopped using the phrase 'hospital bed,' because the connotation is that it's 'end of life' having a medical bed in the lounge room. My discussions with patients when talking about beds was always to focus on the positives, what the electric functions were enabling them to do e.g., to support independence in transfers, to help them sleep better etc.

I have put a lot of thought into how you approach the patient, the words I use and what means the most to them.

Tell me about a situation where you felt you had a great impact?

There are so many. I still have people that reach out to me 10 years later, on the anniversary of a loved one's death just to say hello.

I can think of a couple of people that have a special place in my heart.

Recently there was a gentleman from Melbourne who had developed neurological symptoms during COVID-19. Melbourne had an incredibly long lockdown period over several years. So, coming out of that we were seeing people quite symptomatic in terms of patterns of weakness or speech. They were ending up in our hospital because things had fallen apart at home. We were really playing a lot of catch up with these patients.

One year, this gentleman spent Christmas by himself in hospital, he felt so isolated and lonely. He got discharged but subsequently was diagnosed with motor neurone disease and ended up back in hospital about eight weeks before Christmas for the second year running. His family were dealing with his diagnosis, he was already needing to use a power wheelchair and could not walk at all. So, I did a visit to his house only to find it had ten steps at the front door. Of course, there was no way to make a ramp, and they didn't have any money. I ended up finding a solution through sheer determination - a vertical platform lift from a company that normally uses them for stage shows or concerts. I convinced the owner of this company to loan one to me so this guy could get home to his family for Christmas. I was very persuasive, and we got some help through charitable funding so that was a great outcome.

I do a lot of technology adaptations for people. Setting up devices for people and then experiencing the communication pour out of them when they figure out how it all works, it's so valuable.

The client I spoke of earlier with flail upper limb, motor neurone disease and his smoking aid - it was very satisfying to see him get home. Then we got him back on the computer using some technology and he just perked up, he could get back online with his children. Before the diagnosis he had been the one that cooked in the house and now his wife had had to start cooking. He was so happy to still be part of the process by choosing the meals and doing the grocery shopping online. It made him feel he had some purpose and some role back in his world.

I have a long list of amazing stories, so many great experiences - I still feel it's such a privilege to do what I get to do.

What's your ambition for the future of yourself, for OT and for your patients?

Recently the OT Manager position came up at the hospital and most people thought I was going to apply for it. However, I realised that my skill set is best used when I am patient-facing and helping with student education and supervising juniors. I really don't have an interest in budgets and spreadsheets, so I know that a senior management role is not for me.

A couple of years ago I was invited to start teaching at one of the universities as a sessional academic even though I have no postgraduate qualifications. A couple of times a year I do an intensive module on assistive technology, and I have really been enjoying that. That said, I definitely don't want to be an academic, I don't want to do a PhD or carry out research. What I do really love is teaching students about the reality of being an OT, that's what I bring to those fourth-year units.

You have a hypothetical patient on paper, but that's a very one-dimensional case study, I want to bring the whole person to the discussion and discuss with them what it's like in the real world. I currently have a fourth-year student with us for eight weeks and I want to do more of that - get more of them out to work to gain experience.

I am working more with the Motor Neurone Disease Association of Australia, and The International Alliance and both have been really thrilling to be involved with. I'm really enjoying the international collaboration aspect of it. For example, I'm involved with a couple of therapists from America and we're looking at how we change the narrative for therapists.

I've never really planned out my career, it just kind of happens. As long as I'm doing a good job, the feedback is good and I still feel like I'm learning and growing, then I think at the moment, I'll just continue doing what I'm doing.

I think that's very admirable; you're doing some very valuable things there. One, you are training students - that's very impactful. Two, you are promoting and advancing the care for MND and all neurological conditions. I am impressed with the international collaboration to advance the care of the patients, that's critical.

What to you is the Power of OT?

Many years ago, I read this quote, and it has stuck with me, as it is how I would like someone to describe my input with people.

'Medicine adds days to life. But Occupational Therapy adds life to days.'

This is especially important when working with those with motor neurone disease who have very limited days, it just really hits home the importance of quality of life in every day.

Is there was one thing you would like to see done differently in OT or that you would like to transform?

It would be around that dignity of risk. I've felt it over the last few years, maybe it's because I'm a bit older and maybe because my Risk Barometer has gone down. But certainly, I feel that therapists are becoming more prescriptive and less creative. That might be due to time pressure, funding pressure, differences in supervision.

'I talk to my students and my grads about the 'Nana test.'

Are you treating this client how you would want your nana, or your grandpa or your mum or your dad to be treated?

Are you providing the input that you would like for someone you love?'

I always just come back to the fact that everyone is different. And there's often no clinical pathway for what we're doing. We must keep these people at the centre of what we're doing. I think that the beauty of OT is that in our profession we can truly have an impact on so many areas of someone's life. We must never lose that.

Martina's Key Takeaway: We need to be sensitive with the words we use. Words are powerful. The wrong words used carelessly can cause harm, lower self-esteem and cause emotional pain. However, the right words spoken timely have the power to educate, inspire, motivate and heal.

"It is the activities that we engage in on a day to day basis that make us who we are."

Shoshanah Shear

9

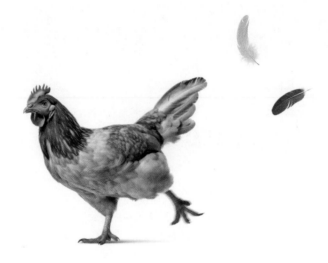

Chicken Run

Kate Sheehan

Fellow of the Royal College of Occupational Therapists (RCOT)
Member of the World Federation of OT
Director, The OT Service

England

'I was working in East London where there were still lots of outdoor toilets, no heating and houses were generally in poor condition.

I saw the impact that poor housing had on the disabled person or someone with a stroke trying to use an outdoor bathroom. That's when I got my passion for housing.'

Kate has been someone whom I have admired from a distance for many years. She has been very influential in the OT world, and she came to mind very early on when I was planning this project on The Power of OT. When I sat down to talk to Kate, I discovered we had a lot in common. We started our private work at much the same time and some of our experiences mirrored each other. It was a pleasure to discover more about her during our chat.

Kate is a Director of The OT Service, a private practice offering expert OT assistance and guidance, and a leading Occupational Therapist in home modifications for people with disabilities.

Just to get started can you give me an idea of your current role and how your business operates?

I have my own private business which I share with Lucy Leonard, Adam Ferry and Samantha Shann. It's a private practice and we cover four areas.

1. We work with companies on product development and writing relevant clinical documentation to support promotion of their products. We have worked with various healthcare equipment manufacturers but also other companies outside of the disability sector, e.g., bathroom solutions companies.

2. We work with people who have had catastrophic injuries, providing rehabilitation and housing solutions.

3. We work with local authorities completing specialist housing assessments and providing expert review on complex case reviews.

4. Finally, we are increasingly providing assessment and adaptation recommendations to private clients who are on waiting lists and cannot access services in a timely manner.

Working with private clients is increasing but much of my work is with catastrophic injuries where there is a medical legal claim and expert OT input is required. This may involve housing adaptations, rehabilitation or specialist equipment needs. It covers everything. What I love about that area of work is that I can truly be an Occupational Therapist. If we can justify it, we are not restricted by the type of equipment we can give, the advice we can share, or the housing we can provide.

Can you tell me about any interesting cases you've worked with?

Yes, there are so many interesting cases - I think that's the other bonus of working in the private sector, I've known some of my clients for decades.

I would like to tell you about two clients. One is an adult; the other is a child.

The first one is a young lady who was involved in a road traffic incident and sustained a spinal injury. I met her when she was at Stoke Mandeville Hospital on bedrest. They were trying to stabilise her back at the time. I was just getting to know her and like most OTs, my first question was 'What do you want to do?'

She said, 'I want to be able to ski with my two-year-old daughter.'

It was a huge challenge. I said, 'OK, that's the goal, but where do we start?'

So, we literally started at the beginning. We went through the process of trying to get her home into a suitable property. Her flat was on the 4th floor with no lift. We first got her into a rental property and then I worked with her to find her forever house. She was very specific about her requirements e.g., it had to be near a school where she could wheel her daughter to school and bring her back home again. The school itself had to be accessible as well as the house and the community she was living in.

With a lot of these legal cases, they are eventually settled and the clients themselves often then sack everyone. I think that's a positive thing because until then, they have been managed to the nth degree. They are being advised by Physios, OTs, Speech and Language Therapists, Psychologists and there comes a time where some people just need all the therapists to go away. They want to take back control.

So, she came to me and said, 'I'm really sorry, I'm sacking everyone.' Then, three months later she came back again and said, 'I need your help.' She wanted to go back to work. Once we got her back to work, she said 'I'm going to sack you again!'

Another while later she called me and said, 'I want to learn to ski.' I knew she was perfectly capable of organising this herself, so

I put her in touch with the SnowDome indoor ski training centre at Milton Keynes - she didn't need me to do it for her. About a year later I got a text, and it was a picture of her in Verbier ski resort in Switzerland with her daughter.

I didn't do everything to get her to that point, she did most of it herself, but the Power of OT is to give people the thought that they can achieve what they want to achieve and do what they want to do. Of course, there will be hurdles but there are often ways of getting over those barriers if that's truly what they want to do.

I have another excellent example. A recent client of mine is an eight-year-old girl who sustained a catastrophic injury at birth. She has cerebral palsy and is nonverbal. When I first met her, I was instructed to look at housing. But, as I sat with this young girl, I saw that everything was happening around her, people were talking and chatting. I looked into her eyes and thought 'She knows what's going on, but she is obviously finding it difficult to communicate.'

We got the Speech and Language Therapist involved to get her a communication device and I was involved in making her home accessible. We worked out that if we got the right chair with the strips on the floor, she could take herself wherever she wanted to go. Just about six weeks ago I went back to see how she was managing the chair and navigating around the house. We were chatting away on the communication device because she was now able to communicate. Then she just said, 'Bye-Bye Kate.' She had had enough. She switched on her wheelchair and went out to the garden. To me the power of being able to communicate what we want is so important and for once being dismissed felt really great!

Are you still involved with the RCOT Specialist Group for Housing?

Yes, I'm now Vice-Chair of the RCOT-SS Housing*. The specialist section is very powerful, and it has had huge amounts of influence in central government and although we are only getting little wins, all those little wins add up. Engaging with government, civil servants and politicians on all sides is key to getting housing designed suitably but we still have got a long way to go.

What would you like to see in the future in terms of housing for people with disabilities?

I would like to see homes designed and refurbished so that they're accessible but do it in an aesthetic way, so people don't feel that they are being given something that is 'white and plastic' or which appears institutional and clinical. We need to create a built environment that allows people to engage and that's not just people with disabilities, it's mums or dads with buggies or students with a bicycle, so that you can use your home as a home. We need to remove those built environmental barriers, that's equality.

Regarding housing, what has been achieved that has been very transformative?

One thing that has been achieved by RCOT-SS Housing is raising the profile of OT within housing, we are being listened to now. Another massive achievement is that the UK Government Department of Levelling Up, Housing and Communities will come to us and ask for our advice and that's across all political parties.

*The RCOT has many special interest sections, where specialists in a subject area come together in sub-groups to share experiences and drive best practice. E.g., RCOT-SS Housing is a special interest group for housing. This section has now been closed as RCOT are reimagining their communities.

We have lobbied for, and we hope this government will agree, to all new-build houses being designed as 'Category 2.' This means that they are adaptable for people with disabilities, they're not designed for people with disabilities, but they have features that will enable them to be used. e.g., Level access, larger accessible ground floor toilets, space for storage, which is always lacking, the kitchen designed with easy adaptation in mind, stair layouts which are suitable for a stairlift, the lounge designed to accommodate a through floor lift if required. Simple things that don't impact cost on the initial build but provides a good standard of housing if adaptation later becomes a requirement.

Who do you need to influence for that to become a standard?

We influence the politicians and the civil servants. The way in is through the civil servants. Give them your time. When they ask a question, I always say 'Let's go for a coffee,' because you can get across so much more over a coffee than through emails. We build up those relationships, network with people and eventually those networks then allow you to say, 'I need to speak to somebody else about this.' With personal introductions it is much more likely you will be listened to and can influence change.

'Never, ever miss an opportunity to speak to a politician! That's how we can influence and change things.'

Can we go back a few years and tell me why you chose OT as a career?

I didn't receive very good careers advice at school. At 14 the careers advisor said, 'You are very caring so you could be a doctor or a nurse... but since you are not bright enough to be a doctor, I think you should be a nurse.' Not very kind advice!

Around that time my father had a family visit us from Australia where the wife was an OT. She spent the weekend telling me how amazing Occupational Therapy was, so I went back to school on Monday and said, 'I'm going to be an OT!'

They said they had no idea what that was, but that I could go find out about it for myself. That Australian lady really opened my eyes to the profession - in the end I was the only one in my class who chose to study Occupational Therapy.

Tell me about your early years as an OT.

When I first trained, I wanted to work in mental health, that was always my area of interest, but I decided to start with a physical rotation. We were privileged back then to have a Basic Grade Rotation where we had the luxury of trying several rotations in different specialisms to find what suited us best.

There were lots of posts for OTs, so I went to London. I had lived in Manchester my whole life and I thought it would be cool to work near the Houses of Parliament! Back then it was easy to get a job - there was no interview, no application process.

St. Thomas's Hospital was opposite the Houses of Parliament, so I simply called them one day and asked if there were any jobs available. The Head OT said 'Yes, when would you like to start?' and that was that!

After the Basic Grade Rotation, I moved back to Derby to do a Senior 2 rotation which included a great mix of physical and mental health. This included Orthopaedics, Care of The Elderly, Burns and Plastics, and Acute Psychiatry.

I still was not sure what area I wanted to work in, so I returned to London to earn some money as a locum as I planned to go travelling. However, I met my future husband, who also worked in London and that ended my impulse of travelling at that time.

It was the early 1990s at that point and I applied for a job in social services with the local authority. I was working in East

London where there were still lots of outdoor toilets, no heating and houses were generally in poor condition. I saw the impact that poor housing had on the disabled person or someone with a stroke trying to use an outdoor bathroom. That's when I got my passion for housing.

> **'I suddenly realised that regardless of your impairment or disability, whether it's physical, mental health or cognitive, your home is key to everything! It impacts hugely on your physical and mental well-being.'**

How important was the Basic Grade Rotation post?

I think that rotation post was so vital as it gave the graduates the foundations for practice. Many local authorities who have links with the universities are offering rotations again now to encourage people to come and work for them because there is still a shortage of OTs. It allows the graduate to find out about themselves, where they can give the best to the patient and find personal and professional fulfilment.

What led you to the decision to move away from your job and go into private practice?

It happened by accident. I'd like to say it was a plan, but it wasn't at first. A friend asked me if I would do some moving and handling training for a client of hers who had come back from Australia. They had a compensation package and wanted new carers trained. At first, I refused to do it, I hadn't thought about private practice, however she kept insisting and I did it just to help her out. When I completed the training, I realised it offered me so much opportunity, so I did another case and then another. I decided to reduce my hours in my local authority job and continued to develop my private practice.

In December 2000 I had an interesting interaction with my manager. I requested to change my days for that week so that I could go to my son's school nativity play. When my request was declined it made me reflect on priorities and work-life balance. At that time my children were young, and I wanted to be there for them so that's when I left my job and went full-time into private practice.

You said you were very hesitant to go into private practice initially - did you feel there was a stigma around private practice at that time?

Yes, I felt like others judged my decision and I was made to feel like a pariah. My first piece of private work was in 1995, and I had so many comments from so many people about 'going to the dark side,' and asking, 'How can you charge for your professional services?'

I thought this was strange because we were all being paid in the NHS and social care; they too were being paid for their professional service. It was very difficult at times to try and explain to people why I was doing it.

As a private practitioner we still use our clinical knowledge, adhere to the Code of Conduct and make ethical decisions based on the needs of the client and carers. In fact, many times in private practice we are even providing an enhanced service because we have more time, we are able to look at the whole person. We are not restricted on what help we can offer or what equipment we can provide.

What I enjoyed initially in private practice and still to this day, is that you can stop and think. You're not on a treadmill. You can sit with your clients and if today is not the right day for them to talk or do a particular assessment then we can do it again another day. In the NHS or social services, you don't always have that luxury of time.

Has the perception of private OT changed, and would you recommend it for anyone considering that path?

Yes, I believe it has changed hugely now in the UK.

'OTs now have more of what I would call a 'portfolio career."

They might do some work in social care alongside some private work, or NHS with private work. They might do work in the third sector maybe in a charity, social enterprise or other community organisation. OTs are now more willing to have a wider experience which is a positive step because each part benefits from the other. Private practitioners are now seen in a much better light. In the UK there may be an underlying negative attitude towards a healthcare professional getting paid privately for their services, some people may ask 'Is it ethically, right?' But we pay for lawyers, plumbers and many other people with experience so why would we not do this in the health sector when it can have a profound and positive effect on someone's quality of life?

As a private practitioner I feel that I can go over and above to give the best service. I do weekend visits. If we are looking at personal care, I would be in there at 7am in the morning or if somebody works and they need a 6pm appointment I can accommodate that too. I can be more flexible and not restrained by a service provision.

Can you tell me about a memorable experience with a patient that really impacted you?

The first was a lady in her early 50s was who involved in a road traffic collision. She was hit by another driver who accidentally put her foot on the accelerator instead of the brake resulting in a spinal injury. She ended up in hospital just before the pandemic and was still there during COVID-19. I went to see her in hospital, we were just chatting and I said, 'What do you want to do?'

She burst into tears. We were in a six bedded room, so it was very difficult to have a private conversation, but I pulled the curtains round and asked if she was ok. She said,

'You are the first person in six months to ask me what I want to do.'

The answer was that she wanted to be able to feed her chickens when she got home but had no idea how she would be able to do that with the limitations she now had. She rescued chickens and had about 20 of them! These poor homeless chickens came to her looking sad and without feathers, but she said she loved caring for them and watching their feathers grow back. Her goal was to be able to feed them, let them out of the chicken coop in the morning and get them back in in the evening to make sure they were safe from the foxes. She also wanted to get back to sitting next to them because she said they all had little personalities and used to jump on her lap like a cat for her to stroke them!

So, we got to work. Like any OT process we graded it and we worked out what we had to do to be able to achieve the goal. It wasn't easy, she lived in a lodge which was a Grade II listed building 'of special interest'* and every effort had to be made to preserve it. It was in the middle of nowhere with a garden on different levels. So, we had to relocate the chickens to an accessible level, and would you believe that we actually found automated

There are UK protection laws to preserve the integrity of older buildings or those with historical significance. This can have a major impact on any modifications or adaptations and the level of protection is graded: Grade I – buildings are of exceptional interest; Grade II – particularly important buildings of more than special interest; Grade II – buildings that are of special interest.

coop openers? I never thought I would need to know that!

We worked out that if we installed a camera with voice control she could 'cluck' at her chickens and the chickens would think she was by her coop and go in. She counted the chickens then she would press a button, and the coop door would close again. She could do it all again in the morning. We created a little space next to the coop where she could wheel in with her wheelchair and her chickens would come and jump on her. It's amazing where OT can take you!

For most people looking on, it might not seem like an important goal, even a strange goal. However, for her to know she was going to be able to return to doing what she was able to before her accident had such a positive impact. We can't underestimate the value of what we did for that lady and many more like her.

She said 'I can now sit and stroke my chickens. I feel my blood pressure going down and I can feel the joy coming back.'

'Without that goal I'm not sure I would have wanted to come out of hospital.'

I have lots of memories and stories from through the years, but one funny example was when I was a brand-new OT. I was so proud of my new green trousers – it was the Occupational Therapy uniform at the time.

Back then when someone was going to be discharged home from hospital, the OT used to pack all the equipment into their car and take the patient home to see whether they would be able to manage.

It was time for my first of these discharge assessments. I took an elderly gentleman to his home as I had been told by the physiotherapist that he could manage to go upstairs. We got halfway up the stairs, and he said with a hint of panic in his voice, 'I can't go any further.'

So, I thought quickly and put my knee against his buttock and said, 'That's OK, just perch on my knee for a moment, have a rest, take a breath and then we'll see whether we should turn round or continue upstairs.'

He simply said, 'I'm really sorry.' For a moment I didn't know what he was sorry for until I felt the warmth of urine going down my legs and into my shoes! The poor man was mortified.

'It's fine, don't worry about it, these things happen!' I said. It had certainly never happened to me before, but I was trying to put him at ease. We returned to the ward and got the patient comfortable, all the while he was constantly apologising. I distinctly remember squelching back into the OT department.

'My lesson from that day was you can never plan for everything and always have a change of clothes!'

Did you have any early role models or anyone who has really encouraged you in your profession?

There were lots of people but the first person who really inspired me was my Head OT in social services, Ruth Ball. She was so passionate about housing and so good at teaching skills. She was the person who taught me to do scale drawings, to understand building construction and she was one of those people who said, 'You know, you can go anywhere.'

Another person who inspired me but in a slightly different way was Diana, she was the Head OT at the Royal Borough of Windsor and Maidenhead local authority outside London. When I had been working there for three months, she took me aside and said, 'I don't think statutory services is your thing. I think you've got potential to do other things.' I questioned her because until that point I had wanted to someday become the Director of Social Services. She said, 'You've got skills outside of this, you'll do something different.'

Sometimes life takes you on a journey which maybe you had not planned. At this time, I was part of the RCOT-SS Housing, and I was invited to an RCOT social drinks event where a colleague introduced me to a man called Tony. He worked for a well-known bathroom manufacturer and had been sent to the event by his boss.

My opening words were 'Can I talk to you about toilets?' and we proceeded to have a full conversation about bathroom fixtures and the problems with their design. We talked about toilets, wash hand basins, showers, baths and at the end of it we exchanged contact details. Two weeks later he rang me and said, 'We are going to do a project called 'Designing Well for Older People, would you like to be involved?' That chance conversation about toilets kick-started my consultancy work with major companies. So, I would say that Tony influenced me as well. He was not an OT but what he had was passion. He said, 'You introduced me to OT, and I introduced you to manufacturing.'

I strongly believe that partnership is key to getting functional and aesthetic design right.

As OTs we tend to focus a lot on toilets… Once, I went to Sydney for the World Federation of Occupational Therapy conference, and as I was wandering around Darling Harbour one evening I noticed they had these amazing, accessible toilets. I was mesmerised! So, I was there trying to hold the door open and trying to take photographs from lots of different angles.

A policeman came along and said, 'What on earth are you doing?!'

When I explained my deep passion for toilets he just walked off, shaking his head. I suppose it must have seemed a little strange!

What would you say is the Power of OT?

As I approach my sixtieth birthday I have been reflecting a lot recently; What is it about OT that I love? It's the kindness.

It's giving the client a chance to talk, and to be listened to, and repeat back what it is that they want.

I was always told at college that you shouldn't get emotionally involved with your clients but looking back, I would challenge that now. I honestly believe that you can't really understand your clients unless you form some element of attachment. Yes, you must be able to walk away from it, but at the same time the emotion helps you to work with your client collaboratively.

When I started my training in 1983, I didn't really understand the profession or see where it was going to go. Now I know we can go anywhere.

'If I could do it all again, I would do so in a heartbeat.'

Martina's Key Takeaway: The only limitation to OT is our imagination. We can work with a client, we can be service providers, we can work with manufacturers, we can work with and in education, we can work with government. There are no limitations to what you can do. To me that is so positive.

"I enjoy the pace, the variety of diagnoses, and the level of complexity of patients in the acute setting. I also feel like there is greater opportunity to see and learn from other disciplines, which helps me grow as a therapist."

David S. McGuire

10

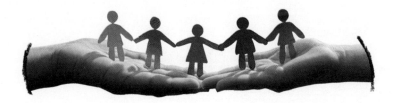

Equity, Diversity and Belonging

Odeth Richardson

Head Occupational Therapist, Newcastle Upon Tyne Hospitals
Chair of Council, Royal College of Occupational Therapists

England

'We need to get into schools to start
to speak to students when they're young.
We need to educate on the value of the
OT profession when they are considering
their course options at university
application stage.'

M y first encounter with Odeth Richardson was at an
RCOT conference in Edinburgh where I was invited to
speak to a specialist interest group of private practitioners. Her
reputation as a leader in our profession is well recognised by her
peers and her determination and desire to transform the profession
is as welcomed as it is refreshing.

It's not easy to take that step and put yourself forward
for change because it's always a challenge to be the first to do
anything. The profession needs people who are willing to push
the boundaries and keep it up to date and in line with social and
cultural changes.

I felt it was important to include Odeth's views in this
book as she is a proponent of much needed change and it was very
interesting to listen to her viewpoint and hear her vision for the
future.

Can we start by asking where did you train to be an OT and why did you come into the profession in the first place?

I completed my training at Brunel University in London in the year 2000. I first came across Occupational Therapy in one of the large teaching hospitals in London, where I was working as a healthcare assistant in theatres at the time. I was sent up to the ward to collect a patient for theatre. This is where I first came across OTs and I was fascinated by their interventions and approach to the patients. I took a few minutes to ask them a few questions: 'What are you doing, and what profession is this?' I had never heard of Occupational Therapists up until that point, but I decided then that I was going to have a look at OT as a career. I suppose you could say I came upon it almost by accident.

That's interesting, where did you start your career?

When I was training to be an OT, I had several placements. The one that stood out for me most was my final placement in Harrow social services in Greater London. I knew then that I wanted to work in the community in local authority because I was fascinated with the variety of adaptations and being able to adapt the environment to make a difference in people's lives. But I also knew having listened to other OTs that it was important to have a varied foundation at the beginning of your career to be able to draw upon different experiences.

So, instead of going directly into social services, I opted to do a Basic Grade post with several rotations: one in neurology; one in older people's medicine; and one in mental health.

When I finished my rotations, I went to work in Harrow social services for a few years and from there I transferred to another service in nearby Brent. After that I moved to Newcastle upon Tyne in the northeast of England where I went back into the acute hospital setting. I have spent half my career in social services and half in acute hospitals.

And what is your role there now?

My role is Operational Manager, I am responsible professionally for the Occupational Therapists across the health trust. I am professional lead as we have some OTs who sit within our community services who are operationally managed by nurses. I provide professional support for them as well as the OTs who work within the acute services.

How many OTs do you have responsibility for at the moment then?

It's a large team of 120. I think it's very important for people to get to meet and get to know each other so we try to have in-person meetings as often as possible. Sharing ideas is such an important part of our work, and we can do that much easier when we're face to face.

Tell me about your role as Chair of Council of the Royal College of Occupational Therapists. It sounds very interesting.

Yes, it is interesting. I am in my second year now. Within the RCOT we've got very unusual governance arrangements, so the role of chair is appointed on a yearly basis during the annual meeting in June. Each year you must reapply for that role, whereas the role of Council member is appointed every three years.

I fell into the role as I always felt I was on the outside of the profession looking in. For years I've been a member of the RCOT but just didn't feel part of the organisation. Following the death of George Floyd, I started looking at the profession and reflected 'We could potentially be a little bit more diverse.'

I also believe we could do a bit more for our members. I was one of those people when the ballot papers come through the door, I'll look at it if I recognise someone, then I'll probably vote for them. But I didn't really take a keen interest in terms of what the profession was doing. Then I thought, well, I can't sit back and complain that the profession isn't doing this or that, I need to do my part. When the role of Chair came up, I looked at it and thought I haven't been on any of the regional boards for a while, but I had a lot of transferable skills having sat as Chair for some other charities within the Northeast of England. I also do some work with Northumbria Police as part of their strategic Independent Advisory group. I spoke to the RCOT CEO Steve Ford and Diane Cox, who was the Chair at the time, just to see what the role entailed and to see if my skills would be transferable to support this role. They said yes, I submitted my form, and I was voted in. I think for the first time there were two or three people who were interested in that role. Normally, the Chair role is the most difficult to fill. So hopefully when I hand over the baton to somebody else, it might encourage more OTs to put themselves forward to be part of this role.

Can you reapply for that role year on year or is there a limited time in which you can hold that post?

There is a limited time in which I can hold it. Now, I'm in my second year and I have applied for a third year. There are things I want to complete before my tenure is over. We've started the governance review as it is outdated. For example, it doesn't really make sense to have a Chair in a role for one year, whereas the rest of council is in place for three years. The other challenge is that a lot of our council members have been appointed at the same time, therefore we have four or five who will be stepping down at the same time. That puts the organisation at risk. We lose that knowledge all at once so that's the reason why I decided to reapply for another year.

The role of Chair has been an interesting one. It has been eye-opening in terms of how the organisation is run and the improvements we can make. I went into the role slightly naïve. I wanted the member's voice to be better heard as I felt it was lost within the professional body. I have campaigned to get them re-engaged and to make sure the members' voices are heard. Their disengagement with the profession was something that really troubled me. One of my staff said to me. 'I don't vote for council members because I don't know anybody. So long as I'm getting my insurance covered by the profession, that's all I need.'

I think that's a sad state as so many members have so much to offer. So that re-engagement piece is very important for me.

What made you feel that you were outside of the profession looking in?

When I looked at all the communication that was coming out of RCOT, it was very white, and I didn't see anybody that looked like me within the profession. With the structures and systems we have in place I just felt that it wasn't for me. Occupational Therapy looked like one of those very white, middle-class professions. It is also very female dominated and so we haven't really done a lot in terms of adding diversity.

When I look at the current strategy, I thought for the first time it was something I could identify with because there were parts of it that really spoke to me. We are gradually moving forward, and this is something that I can champion.

Can you tell me about an experience that stands out where you felt you had great impact?

When I worked in social services, I had a young man who had been on holiday and dived into a pool. The pool was too shallow, and he suffered a spinal injury resulting in quadriplegia. When he came home, I needed to make sure that his home was suitable so that he could do the things that were important to him as a young man and to be able to live a fulfilling life. This was one of the best adaptations I have done. I was able to put things in place to make sure that he had his own private space at his home and a place where he was able to use all the environmental controls to support him to become independent. I knew I had done a good job because of the gratitude from his parents and from the young man himself. As OTs we advocate for our clients, and we can do things to make a difference to enhance their quality of life. So, to me that always stood out as one of my greatest achievements. To enable him to live life to the maximum.

Did you ever find yourself in a situation where you felt OT was not valued and if so, what did you do about it? Or how did you feel about it?

Yes. Within the acute hospital setting, in my experience multidisciplinary team members look to OTs to arrange discharge from the hospital as soon as possible to make more beds are available - OTs are at times considered to be discharge planners. However, what they miss is the value that Occupational Therapy brings to our patients. Sometimes we as OTs are our own worst enemies in that when we're in those MDT situations or on ward rounds, we don't use the language of occupational science to demonstrate what we bring to the table. When I identified that within my own service, we did a lot of work with the team around the language we use to demonstrate the impact we can have and the difference we can make. As OTs we need to go back to basics.

When people come into hospital, some of them can be occupationally deprived because their regular life stops sometimes suddenly, and they are in a strange environment. OTs need to recognise this in patients, remove the occupational deprivation and try to enhance their stay so that they can then go home and live fulfilled lives. It is starting to change but because of the quick turnover of medics and nursing staff who rotate very often we are constantly having to retrain staff in the acute setting about our role and where we fit in.

Have you big aspirations of where you would like to see the profession going?

We've just completed our workforce strategy and we have identified a significant shortage of OTs nationwide.

> 'I would like to see our apprenticeship programme really take off.
> There are many OT Assistants and Technical Instructors who are highly skilled but have not had the opportunity to get trained to become qualified OTs.
> They are the next generation of OTs.
> It's my goal is to try and invest in this cohort of people.'

We do have international recruitment, but we are limited to how many people we can bring in. It's very important that we start to grow our own OTs. We need to get into schools to start to speak to students when they're young. We need to educate on the value of the OT profession when they are considering their course options at university application stage. I believe we're not very good at that. That's something that we really need to focus on over the next few years. We need to work together to raise the profile of OT and also continue to lobby government as well.

That's something that really speaks to my heart. I'm nearing the end of my career and sometimes it's only on reflection that you look back and see the benefit of the career and the impact you've had, not only on your patients, but only also on yourself and on your own family. That's something that I am really passionate about - it's one of the reasons I'm writing this book and talking to you today. I want to capture the attention of the students early on, when they are thinking about applying to university.

What in your opinion, is the value and the Power of OT?

We have a group of retired OTs and I keep in touch with them because they have so many skills and so much knowledge. I think as a profession we don't use that group enough. So, among colleagues I keep pushing to say, 'We have this skill set here, with a fabulous wealth of knowledge, we really need to engage with that group.'

We need to make sure that we're helping that hard-earned expertise pass down through generations. Retirees also feel disenfranchised by RCOT because they feel their voice isn't being heard. We are now listening. We need to engage with them to see how we can use their expertise.

'You never quite retire from OT.'

OT can make such a difference to people at any stage of their life, from birth through to death, we can make a difference. We can help enhance the quality of life for our patients. The Elizabeth Casson lecture says, 'Now is our time.'

We need to start shouting from the hilltop, coming together collectively. Individually, we all have a part to play, but with our collective voice, when we start to work together then together we're stronger.

There is such a variety of things that you can do within OT. There is no end to it. It is one of those professions where you need to find your passion and then you can do anything with that.

'We don't focus on the things
that clients can't do. We focus on the
things that clients want to do within the
limitations that they may have.
That's the skill set that we have.'

Martina's Key Takeaway: Diversity within OT brings a wealth of perspectives, fostering innovation and creativity by blending different ideas and experiences. It promotes a more inclusive and respectful environment and encourages cultural understanding and reduces prejudice, leading to a more equitable society.

"Occupational Therapy practitioners
ask, 'What matters to you?'
not, 'What's the matter with you?'"

Virginia "Ginny" Stoffel

11

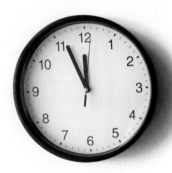

Making a Difference
Takes Time

Kate McWilliams

Occupational Therapy Technician/Assistant
NHS

Northern Ireland

'Job satisfaction for me comes from seeing the positive impact of my work, whether it's providing the right equipment or simply spending time with a patient. I get joy from my work when I solve a problem and see that I've made life a bit easier for the patient or the family.'

It must be recognised that the role of the Occupational Therapy Technician (OTT) or Assistant (OTA) is a vital part of the OT team. An experienced and well-trained OTT provides significant support to the Occupational Therapist, allowing them to focus on assessment and treatment of more complex cases. They also help orientate and guide students and newly qualified staff. I believe that further and specific training of the OTT is an improvement that could allow them to move from being a technician to becoming an Occupational Therapist if they have that desire. Kate has been an OTT for 18 years and plays a key role within her department. She is a constant and reliable member of the team and gave me so much more insight into her role during our interview.

Why did you choose OTT as a career?

My interest in this field was sparked by personal experiences within my family, where I saw the impact of illness and the role of OTs in helping patients. The person-centred approach of OT appealed to me, as it considers the entire person and their environment and I was fortunate enough to secure a position in this field, which I enjoy and find deeply fulfilling. I really feel I can make a difference, for those living with dementia sometimes the difference can be shorter-term and transient but for others it can be lifechanging and long-lasting.

What was your previous experience?

Before becoming an OTT, I was a part-time phlebotomist and I worked in a centre providing day care for the older clients, some of whom had dementia. This gave me many transferable skills which helped me greatly in my new role as an OTT. Prior to that I was a Healthcare Assistant. I've always preferred working with older people because I find their life experiences, knowledge and stories fascinating. I always admire their work ethic and how they have overcome many challenges in their lifetime.

Can you give an overview of your current role and duties?

My current role is within the Occupational Therapy team, where my primary focus is to assist and support the OT. Following an OT assessment of need, a treatment plan is drawn up. My role involves implementation of the plan to help patients regain and maintain independence in their daily living tasks. My approach covers everything from morning routines to bedtime, ensuring that every aspect of the patient's daily life is considered. I assist with various tasks, provide equipment instruct in its safe use and how to safely transfer from bed, toilet, chair, bath etc. I feel that a major part of my role is to support the family and caregivers. As dementia progresses, the focus often shifts from helping the patient to providing more comfort and support to the caregiver, helping them cope with the challenges they face. Sometimes the family may feel overwhelmed and just need someone to talk to. Just today I had a phone call from a family member who was distressed and upset and when the call was over, she said 'Thank you for allowing me to vent.' That's all she needed at that time, someone to talk to. I feel the role of the OTT gives me the opportunity to spend more time with the client and build rapport and a relationship with the family as well as the patient.

'To make a difference takes time. You can't really build a relationship if you are under pressure with time.'

I support the Occupational Therapist in the assessments of patients in the kitchen and when out and about in the community. This will involve accompanying the client to the shops to see how well they manage traffic and lights etc., and how responsive they are to the changing surroundings. This can fluctuate from day to day so needs to be reassessed regularly. I also work with assistive technology, like alarms and switches, to help reduce caregiver stress and improve patient safety. This technology plays a crucial role in helping prevent falls.

How is your caseload allocated and prioritised?

Referrals are allocated based on the specific needs of the patient. Some cases, especially those requiring minor adaptations, can be handled directly by me, allowing for quicker resolution as there is often a waiting list for the OT. I am responsible for ordering and installing rails and other necessary adaptations in patients' homes.

I also have my own caseload, which involves assessing the specific needs of patients. For instance, if a patient needs help with activities like getting on and off the toilet, I conduct a detailed assessment, speak with the family, and determine the most appropriate equipment or interventions. Every six weeks, my caseload is reviewed under supervision which allows me to discuss cases with a senior OT to ensure that I am adhering to the best practices and guidelines. I'm careful to operate within my remit, always checking with an OT if I'm unsure about a particular task or if it should be referred to another member of the team.

'It is important that we are constantly aware of the full picture and not get too focused on one particular intervention.'

I frequently collaborate with social workers, community psychiatric nurses (CPNs), the housing executive, and housing associations.

Continuity of care is crucial, especially in dementia care. I aim to spend as much time as possible with clients and this continuity is so important in my interactions with the MDT, ensuring that all aspects of the person's care are coordinated and effective.

Which parts of your job give you most satisfaction?

Job satisfaction for me comes from seeing the positive impact of my work, whether it's providing the right equipment or simply spending time with a patient. I get joy from my work when I solve a problem and see that I've made life a bit easier for the patient or the family.

Building rapport with patients is essential. I try to remember details from previous visits to show patients and families that I care and to build trust. Convincing patients to use new equipment can be challenging, but I find that taking the time to explain and demonstrate its benefits usually wins them over.

One memorable experience involved a patient with a contracted hand whose skin was at risk of breaking down and who was resistant to using a hand protector. In the beginning she got very agitated and upset and refused to let the OT put it on. I was asked to go out and try again. At first, she remained very resistant but through patience and persistence, I was able to get her to accept the protector, which was crucial for preventing skin damage. It took time. I sat with her and rubbed her hand, I gave her the hand protector to feel, she played with it for a while and held it in her hand eventually I gained her confidence and cooperation. She allowed me to put it on and is still using it.

In addition to community work, I've also worked with groups on the ward for 14 years, where I dealt with some of the more challenging cases, often involving patients whose caregivers could no longer manage them, and homecare had broken down. Group activities like singing and chair-based exercises were effective in engaging patients, even those who were initially reluctant to participate. I had a lady who refused to participate every week; however I was keen to get her involved so each week I went to talk to her, but it was a 'no-go.' After weeks of perseverance, I managed to entice her to join the group. We always ended the group activity with a singsong which she loved. She continued to attend and began to enjoy and look forward to it. When she would see me on the ward, she would come to me and ask when the group was starting!

Do OTTs receive ongoing training and professional development?

I feel that training opportunities for OTTs could be improved. While there is some on-the-job training, I believe there's room for more structured training, we receive the mandatory courses e.g., I receive training on various aspects of patient care, ensuring equipment is set up correctly, moving and handling, but specific additional training for OTTs is rare. We have an OTT forum that meets four times a year, where OTTs from various settings come together to discuss issues and potential training needs. I attend these meetings to stay informed about developments and challenges in the field. This is an area I would like to see more improvement.

Have you ever considered transitioning to OT?

While I have not pursued further education to become an OT, I recognise the potential benefits of additional training and professional development. I believe OTTs would make excellent OTs and more opportunity should be offered to them if they want to pursue a career in OT. Depending on the region and available programs there may be opportunities for OTTs to transition into OT roles. Although this has not been a focus for me, I acknowledge the value it could bring for others.

Do you feel your role as the OTT is valued by others?

I feel my role as the OTA is highly valued within my team. I provide continuity and stability, being a constant presence even as other colleagues come and go and I've been a full-time member of the team for 18 years. My experience and knowledge are often relied upon by new staff and students, which adds to the sense of value in my work. Students accompany me on home visits which gives them a valuable insight into the role. I feel I'm the mainstay of the department and enjoy providing support to the other members of the team.

What do you believe are the key skills and qualities of a good OTT?

I believe to be an effective OTT some key skills include excellent communication, a friendly and empathetic approach, and the ability to work well within a multidisciplinary team, understanding that taking time with patients is vital to develop trust and cooperation. Support and encouragement are key in this role, not just for patients but also for caregivers. Listening to caregivers, understanding their concerns, and offering practical advice can make a significant difference in their ability to cope.

Martina's Key Takeaway: I am reminded of the quote by Joel Osteen, 'The greatest gift you can give someone is your time, your attention, your love, your concern.'

"Man, through the use of his hands,
as they are energized by mind and will,
can influence the state of his own health."

Mary Reilly

12

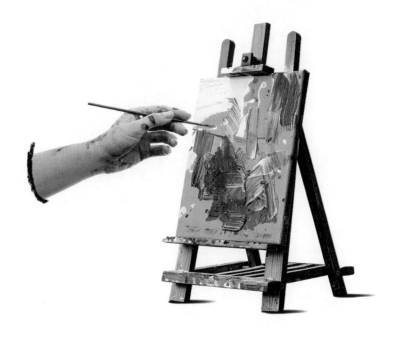

The Art of
Occupational Therapy

Joanne McGowan

*Retired Community Occupational Therapist
NHS & HSE*

Northern Ireland & Republic of Ireland

'Other professions were coming
in and out, concerned about her other
needs such as pressure areas, dressings etc.,
but no one else thought
'Can she take a simple sip of water
when she needs a drink?"

The readers of this book will already be familiar with Joanne as in earlier chapters I mentioned the role she played in helping me establish The Disability Centre and the central role she played at the start of my journey as an Independent OT. I may never have started my journey had it not been for her courage, encouragement and her eagerness to try something new. Joanne's love for her patients and her art propelled her on a different path from when we started in The Disability Centre but as you will read in our conversation it has been very worthwhile and I find her stories inspirational.

Joanne, can you bring me back to the start of your career as an OT?

I started my career as an OT in psychiatry. It was a senior post, but I quickly discovered that working in mental health was not for me. One of the advantages of being an OT is that you can try different aspects of the profession until you find what really suits you. After a year I decided to take a step down in seniority to work as a Basic Grade when a job became available in the geriatric unit of Altnagelvin Hospital. That's where I developed my interest in community OT. In this role, I carried out many home visits to assess the suitability of the home before patients were discharged and I liaised with the community OTs on home adaptations and equipment. After learning to drive, a job vacancy arose in the community, so I decided that's where I really wanted to settle and then I remained a Community OT for 33 years between Derry City and Donegal.

Why did working in the community appeal to you?

When I worked in the day centre, patients were coming in for assessment and treatment, but it was very important to understand their home environment and the challenges they were facing at home. It was not possible to fully rehabilitate someone if we did not have a clear picture and understanding of the family and home environment. At that time the hospital had a van which I could borrow one afternoon each week to carry out the home assessments I needed to do. Seeing a patient only in the clinical setting is not realistic, many homes had very small bathrooms and there were tripping hazards which would increase falls risk. I was really keen to see people in their own homes to see what they could and couldn't do and what we needed to concentrate on in therapy sessions.

In the 1980s many homes were not suitable for people with disabilities. Some homes had no heating, and some did not even have indoor bathrooms. It was often a struggle to make the necessary changes as many patients just wanted to continue living the way they had always done. We needed to be respectful of their wishes but also work closely with them if we felt there were risks involved.

What triggered your interest in Occupational Therapy at the start?

I went to a school where there was very little careers guidance - the only advice was to choose either nursing or hairdressing. I didn't know what I wanted to do but I was thinking about Art College. Art was always my passion but there were few jobs except teaching which involved art and at that time I didn't want to be a teacher. I decided to take a year out to help me make the decision.

Then somebody made a comment to me 'You should do Occupational Therapy, there is lots of arts and crafts in it.' I thought a job involving arts and crafts would suit me so that's how I got interested in it. However, as I hadn't studied a science subject, I had to complete a night class in human biology. I knew very little about OT when I went for my interview and remember being very surprised when I got accepted.

It's ironic that arts and crafts were mainly used in psychiatry therapies and as I have already stated I did not like the mental health role that I had, so I never really used my art skills during my OT career. Now that I am retired, I have at last combined my art skills and my OT skills working as a volunteer in the local Foyle Hospice. The patients love it and so do I.

You didn't fully understand what Occupational Therapy was before you came into it, but do you think it was a good choice for you?

I loved my job as an OT. I enjoyed all my years of work because I loved working with patients. That's actually why I started volunteering in the Foyle Hospice after I retired, because I missed the patient contact. So yes, it was a very good career for me, I loved it.

After leaving The Disability Centre you went to work as a Community OT in Inishowen, a very rural part of Co. Donegal in northwest Ireland. Was this a major adjustment from working as a Community OT in the city? What were the main differences?

There was a big, big difference. The main one for me was that I was so used to the hustle and bustle of the city and everyone being in a hurry. Streets had names, houses had numbers and addresses had postcodes. I arrived in Donegal, there were no landmarks, no Satnav worked there, no postcodes, no names on roads and no house numbers! If I asked for directions people would say things like 'go over the bridge and turn left,' or 'go past the piggery and up the hill for three miles.'

I was looking for a bridge but all I saw was a stone wall which I eventually realised was a bridge! As for what constituted a piggery I was just totally lost! After the first year and learning family nicknames and landmarks around Inishowen it became much easier, by the time I retired with the introduction of Eircodes and Google Maps life for a rural Community OT was a breeze by comparison to those early days!

I grew to love working in rural areas. Having the fabulous landscape of Inishowen to enjoy when I was out and about doing my work was an extra bonus. There was also a cultural difference between the two jurisdictions and between the city and the countryside. The people were totally different as well, I found the expectations of those in the country were much less than the clients I had in the city.

I found that in the city, people expected a lot from the public service, and our service dealt with complaints when their high expectations were not met. When I first arrived in Donegal it was during the Celtic Tiger* years which meant we had access to so much good equipment. Unfortunately, that changed when the economic downturn came in 2009, meaning waiting lists were created or people could buy privately. Either way, clients in Donegal were just so grateful for the assessment and OT intervention. The

* *Celtic Tiger refers to a period of exceptional economic growth and prosperity in Ireland during the 1990s and 2000s*

gratitude I received from them made me feel that I was doing a very worthwhile job.

Tell me about some of the highlights of being an OT, maybe with some patients where you felt that you really made an impact.

I helped one patient who loved to read was living in a nursing home. She was using an electronic book and she was unable to physically push the buttons anymore. I worked with her for a couple of sessions and using a pen with a rubber grip in a certain way we were able to finally get her to push a button. It was the only thing she could do independently, and it meant that she was able to continue reading which improved her life and meant so much to her.

I also remember having a patient with motor neurone disease who needed to summon help at night, but she was unable to do this because she had very little voluntary movement left in her body.

I worked closely with the assistive technology team and between us we devised a switch that fitted inside a glove which she could wear at night to summon help when needed. Because of this she wasn't frightened every night going to bed as she did not feel so isolated.

This same client spent long periods of time on her own and was unable to keep herself hydrated, so again with the help of the assistive technology team we were able to adapt a cup with a straw and mount it onto her tilt in space chair so that she could manage to drink during the day on her own.

It was these small things that were so important. Other professions were coming in and out, concerned about her other needs such as pressure areas, dressings etc., but no one else thought 'Can she take a simple sip of water when she needs a drink?'

Sometimes other professions focus more on the major things which is important of course, but it's often the small things that matter most to the patient and can make the biggest difference to their life.

What is the value to the patient of having an OT?

During my career many of my OT colleagues would get annoyed about the perception of OT being the 'equipment providers.' But I always accepted it as a compliment, because to me the OT is the one person that should be the expert in what equipment is available and should know the equipment inside out. They should have an up-to-date knowledge of what equipment is on the market and available for their patients. So, to me the OT superpower is our knowledge of equipment. I always said to OTs who were starting out in their career,

'Learn the equipment, learn how to use it and make sure that you are the expert in that equipment. If somebody calls you an 'equipment provider,' be proud! That is our job, and no other profession knows the value of equipment like we do or the power that properly assessed and correctly fitted equipment can give to your patient.'

To use equipment properly, you must do an activity analysis. For example, you must analyse how the patient gets in and out of a chair, how they move and what their limitations are. So, you're not just handing out a piece of equipment or a chair or a bath aid, you're looking at how the patient is going to interact with a piece of equipment and that's where the skill comes in as an OT. You are never "just" an equipment provider.

Did you find during your career that you had enough time to spend with your patient, or did you find that you were rushed?

When I was less experienced, I always felt rushed and sometimes the paperwork took priority over patient contact. I know keeping records is very important but as my career progressed, I did try to spend more and more time with patients and prioritise them over administrative tasks. Even as a part-time OT I managed to see many more patients than was expected of me, because that was important. I knew they needed my help, and patients always came first.

Have you ever felt that the role of OT is a little misunderstood?

It is misunderstood. I have felt for a long time that the name Occupational Therapy isn't the right name for our profession. Does it really reflect what we do? It confuses people. Some people ask 'What do you do? Do you keep people occupied?' If someone is severely disabled and they don't have a job, then others are thinking, 'Oh, you're keeping people busy.'

I feel it is misleading and I often had to try to explain our role. We often refer to 'meaningful activity' which is much more accurate to explain what we do. I hope this book helps to define Occupational Therapy and highlight the values we bring to patients.

Who were your role models during your career? Did you have anyone that you looked up to or inspired you?

I always admired Doctor Ailbe Beirne who was one of the geriatricians when I worked in Altnagelvin Hospital. I had as much respect for him as he had for the OT profession, and he thought very highly of OTs. He taught me early on that the most important thing for our patients was encouraging and enabling them to do the simple things, like getting to the toilet themselves, getting out of the chair, turning on their heating. During the ward rounds he was very strict with medical students as well as the other professions. He had no time for highfalutin* answers when he asked about the patients' progress. He was very practical and real and would simply say, 'Can they go to the toilet themselves?' He often kept patients in hospital while the family installed heating systems, as he knew this was essential for their long-term health – I don't think that wouldn't happen nowadays!

I have always tried to emulate that approach with my patients.

You have had a great deal of experience with MND patients. Would you like to tell me something about your involvement with this client group?

While some OTs were hesitant about accepting referrals for recently diagnosed MND patients, I was passionate about the need for early intervention and building rapport early on with the person and the family, so I really loved getting the referrals.

These people often lose their ability to communicate verbally, so I always felt that it was essential to get to know them while they could still communicate more easily with me. I always tried to visit at least once per week to assess the progress and make suggestions for equipment in a considerate and proactive manner.

Change can happen so fast so the patient and their family need to have a good level of trust built up so they will accept equipment and adaptations more readily and gradually as it is needed. The patient with MND has complex needs but no more complex than with other patients, the difference is in the urgency. It's essential that the OT really knows the equipment, when to introduce it into the conversation, how to prepare the patient and the family so that they can grow accustomed to the idea and then accept it when necessary.

I heard of one case where there was a recently diagnosed MND patient and the team arrived with a wheelchair the week

* *Highfalutin is an informal phrase meaning pompous or pretentious. When someone is trying to be serious or important, but in a way that often appears over the top and unnecessary.*

after diagnosis! This wheelchair wasn't needed for months, and the patient and family were not prepared in advance for it. Understandably in this instance the patient and the family had huge trust issues going forward with the whole MDT!

It's also important to liaise and build up a good relationship with the MND society in the area as they can assist with support and equipment provision early on. It is very important that junior OTs get the opportunity to shadow the senior OTs when dealing with complex cases as this is how they will learn to manage and cope with difficult and fast-moving cases.

Did you find working with MND patients stressful?

No, I always liked being there for them at what was a stressful time for them. I knew I could add value with my knowledge and experience of MND. The only stress I experienced was when I was concerned that the equipment which was ordered would not arrive on time - timing is crucial for these patients. Working with them was fulfilling and they appreciated my input and honesty when they needed questions answered.

Where would you like to see the profession going in the future?

I think there should be a specialist OT for MND in each area as there's such a fear of the disease. The Occupational Therapist plays a pivotal role in the management of the condition. They are not only a support to the patient themselves, but the needs of the family are also crucial at this very difficult time because people know how progressive it is and how fast change can happen.

I also think there should be more OTs in preventative medicine. We have one OT in Co. Donegal in Ireland who goes out in the emergency ambulance when there's a fall or for an elderly person. Many times, the intervention of the OT along with medial staff means they can avoid hospital admission by providing appropriate equipment and advice, then doing a follow up visit. So that's an area I think we should be pushing more for in the future.

I also think the OT courses need to reflect more accurately the work that the OT will be doing when they are qualified. I really didn't know what to expect when I came out to work. I soon realised that it was all down to common sense and problem solving. I think bringing OTs into colleges as guest speakers to talk about real-life situations is very helpful to prepare students for the world of work.

What would you say to a student who was thinking about being an OT?

I would tell them that there is real job satisfaction in being able to take a patient from not being able to do things for themselves, through rehabilitation, appropriate equipment provision and/or adaptations to a place where they have regained their confidence and independence and improved their quality of life.

One of the best joys from Occupational Therapy is the teamwork. I worked with Public Health Nurses and Physiotherapists in Co. Donegal who were equally dedicated to their patients. There's a team and you need to work well with the other members, then you get support from each other. For example, we carried out joint assessments to ensure we got the most benefit for the patient, we were not working in isolation. Teamwork is imperative especially with progressive long-term conditions where the situation is constantly changing.

As a Community OT you need to be innovative and having good knowledge of the latest equipment is imperative to give the patient the best outcome. I am very envious now of the current OTs as they have access to so much technology which has the potential to make life much easier for the patient. The old environmental control systems were cumbersome and confusing for the patients. Now 'Alexa' can do most things with so much simplicity, it's great to see!

Technology is transforming Occupational Therapy. So as a student if you are interested in technology and the benefit it brings to people with disabilities, OT is definitely a career that can give you real job satisfaction

Can you sum up the Power of OT?

Occupational Therapy has so many powers, it depends on the area you work in, but for me the power of the Community OT is in being able to envisage a home where someone with a disability or health condition can live as fully and independently as possible. This is achieved by knowing the equipment, knowing the adaptations and knowing good housing design.

Being able to prepare the patient and family for what they might expect in the future is a special thing to do. It's about the OT having the confidence in themselves to know that their contribution is invaluable and always remember that the patient is the most important member of the team.

Martina's Key Takeaway: To get the best outcomes for our patients it will sometimes be necessary to provide equipment which is clinically assessed and professionally fitted and that is a skill and true value for our patient. Be proud of this skill, it is the essence of Occupational Therapy.

"To know even one life has breathed
easier because you have lived.
This is to have succeeded."

Ralph Waldo Emerson

13

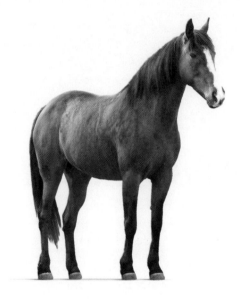

Nature-Based Therapy

Clare McMonagle

Equine Specialist Occupational Therapist
Northern Ireland

'The Power of Occupational Therapy
is your ability to use yourself for
the good of all our people.'

Clare is a busy, dynamic person who has used her OT skills in a unique and resourceful way to help her clients and make the most of the beautiful environment she lives in. She is also a lecturer in Occupational Therapy at Ulster University. Clare lives in a rural area quite close to my home, so I was aware of the special work she was doing in our community. Even for an OT it is progressive and exceptional, but it was not until I sat down to talk to her that I became more aware of the benefits of what she was doing and the remarkable difference she was making to the lives of her clients. Clare is a specialist in equine and nature-based Occupational Therapy, and she also runs a social farm with her family.

Clare, I am very interested to know how you have used your OT skills to develop your own business, can you tell me about it?

I started Gortilea Social Farm in 2014 with the support of my family. As an Occupational Therapist, I was really interested in how we can use the natural environment and the rural resources that we have here to support people that are recovering from mental health issues or people who have learning disabilities. We were initially invited to be involved in a community project for 20 weeks supporting adults with learning disabilities through farm-based activities to gain purposeful employment and add purpose to their day. After the pilot ended, I could really see the benefits for the participants of working alongside my dad, who was the farmer. They gained so much from meaningful work. We received funding to keep it going and we regularly have participants come out to work on the farm alongside my dad and my sister. My sister has a training qualification and provides support for the participants to gain accredited qualifications. As the OT, I help the participants to develop an individualised plan and we utilise the farm and the natural resources to support them to build up to their goals including employment, education and purpose in their day. As part of our farm, we also deliver Equine-assisted Occupational Therapy, which is a more specialist one-to-one area of work and incorporates hippotherapy. We also provide targeted Equine-assisted group sessions when required for young people and children, as well as families.

Why horses? Why hippotherapy?

I've always loved horses. I started riding horses when I was eight or nine years old. I didn't have my own horse as a child, but I just always had a real love for them. My great uncles were interested in horses, and they always understood the power that they had to make you feel better. There is a lot of research available on how beneficial it is, and more and more case studies are coming out involving children who have had their first words and steps during hippotherapy. We have been fortunate to see examples of both first-hand with the clients we have helped.

Tell me more about hippotherapy.

Hippotherapy is the use of the movement of a horse in a treatment session. We use the movement of the horse in a similar way to how you might use a therapy ball or a swing for sensory integration purposes or a balance beam for gross motor activities and coordination. Like any other treatment intervention I follow my OT process, I do the assessment and from that I can see how we could implement the horse. A horse provides 2000 movement inputs per half hour, and I can use that graded movement or input for the child or young person. We also use the ground for the groundwork activities to work on those transferable skills, which will help them in their school environment, at home and in their leisure activities as well.

We also have a therapy room and a mechanical simulator horse. This gives me feedback information about where that child is in terms of their balance and coordination. We use that as a tool to record the progress in weeks one, five and 10. We use a range of standardised assessments when appropriate, including the Movement ABC*, the SCOPE* and the sensory profile. Sometimes the horse is just one element of their therapy sessions, and we also incorporate other elements of intervention, for example we might utilise new lambs or stable management - motivation is key in any successful treatment plan.

We give home plans and strategies for parents and families so it's very much a family-centred approach.

Movement ABC is a paediatric assessment tool which identifies, describes and guides treatment of motor impairment.

The SCOPE is an occupation-focused assessment that determines how a child's volition, habituation, skills, and the environment facilitate or restrict participation.

'I'm a real advocate of the natural environment and how it can be used in therapy at no cost to the family.'

Where did you do your training in hippotherapy?

My undergraduate degree dissertation was in hippotherapy and its benefits. Back then members of the public were invited to an auditorium and we presented our dissertation to them. There was a man in the audience from Derry City Council who listened to the presentation, and he provided me with information on how to apply for funding to enable me to go to America to do the training. So, Gareth, (my husband now, then boyfriend,) came with me and I did my training there. When I came back it was difficult to continue because there was nobody in practice and nobody delivering this treatment. Eventually I got in touch with an OT called Sarah in Co. Cork in Ireland. She was delivering the treatment and was very supportive. I was able to shadow her in some sessions which was very useful and she helped me to set up my organisation.

'Initially we did a pilot with five children who were volunteers. After the five weeks, a nine-year-old boy called Darragh, who was nonverbal said his first words. I have that on video, and it really helped me then to realise that this was something that I needed to do. It was like a vocation for me.'

We are very lucky now that Ulster University are delivering two Master's modules in Equine Facilitated Therapy, similar to the training I did in America. Back then I didn't have the option, I had to go abroad to study as it was the only place delivering the training, but I'm delighted it is available locally now.

How do you get your referrals and what type of clients come to hippotherapy?

For hippotherapy we have a wide range of referrals - some are self-referrals while others are referred from local healthcare systems. The referrals are mainly for children with a wide range of diagnoses. Primarily we work with children with complex physical disabilities, cerebral palsy, children with Down's syndrome and children that have a diagnosis of neurological conditions. We work with children with Autistic spectrum disorder (ASD) or who struggle with their sensory integration. We teach the families techniques that they can use in the natural environment to support their child going forward. More recently following COVID-19 we have worked with children, young people and their families who have been impacted by trauma and mental health conditions. It has been so valuable for me as an OT to see the benefit they can get from our intervention and how we can help them work through their trauma.

Is your intervention recognised by mainstream?

It is beginning to be recognised here in Northern Ireland. My main problem with expansion is that there is a high level of manpower needed to carry out the activities. We have the OT, two side walkers and then the horse, so it is an expensive intervention. We have done much work collecting evidence to support the intervention demonstrating how it helps each child to reach their goals at a much faster rate. So, the benefit outweighs the cost as they reach their goals much earlier. For example, we have children that have come to us with quadriplegic cerebral palsy, they were told they would never be able to sit up straight, and they've left walking with minimal support from our clinic. We also have many children who have talked for the first time. It is attributed to the bond they develop with the horse, together with the sensory input they gain from the open and natural environment and resources. Due to the training and experience I have done over the years I am able to grade the movement appropriately and get the right response, it's just amazing to see the results we can achieve. We now have health boards who are willing to invest in this programme and we have been successful in delivering a number of contracts for the NHS. We have recently delivered a funded programme for children with Multiple Adverse Childhood Experiences (MACE) with very successful outcomes.

How widely available is this treatment throughout the UK and Ireland?

There are a few hippotherapy centres scattered throughout the UK, but not so many. I think the commercial side of running a business is a barrier for many OTs. We are trained in the delivery of treatment but not in running a business. I was lucky to have the support of my family. Running a business can be challenging and risky, we must develop our procedures, obtain the relevant insurance, promote our services, make sure we have enough work to justify the expenses so it's not attractive for everyone.

'However, the benefits are worth it,
and I think we should encourage more
entrepreneurship in OT.

We need to develop the training to include more of the business side and give the OTs the confidence to have a go at business and private work if they're interested in pursuing it.'

The university has added an Innovation and Leadership Module and a workshop module into the undergraduate training. We want to look at a new way of working in terms of Occupational Therapy. Before students complete their undergraduate programme, they will have an awareness of the huge and varied range of opportunities that are available to them by considering private practice and entrepreneurship.

That brings us to Ulster University and your current role as a full-time lecturer. What are the main skills you are bringing to this role?

I really enjoy my role as a lecturer and I like to bring my clinical skills into the classroom. I think it's important for students to get up-to-date and real-life case studies. The modules I coordinate are 'Children, young people and families,' and 'Vocational Rehabilitation,' both of which are very relevant to our social farming activities. It's very valuable to work within the university. I have brought the students out to the farm a few times and we've been to the beach and the forest. I try to encourage them to think about how they can use natural resources, use what we have. We don't always need huge pieces of expensive equipment. The families can go on day trips and consider how they might use what they have in front of them to be able to get some intervention or some input, if that's needed at the time.

    I enjoy the university as it also provides me with the

opportunity to carry out and lead much needed research in my area of interest. We are finishing up a journal article at the minute on the data that I have collected in our social farming programme. The university encourages us to do that. I want to see other OTs delivering nature-based activities including hippotherapy, equine-assisted learning and social farming.

I believe it is invaluable to have therapists like you with lots of 'hands-on' experience lecturing in the university. It must really help prepare the students for the real working environment.

Over the years I have learned by doing, I'm a real active learner and I think it's hard to beat real-life learning. I say to my students 'We always complete our risk assessments.' It's so important, but it's also very important to be able to think on your feet, risk assessment is a process. That's what I always loved about social farming, sometimes we think too linearly about things when actually you need to use a bit of common sense as farmers do. They are risk assessing all the time. I think that's what we do as OTs and that's what I like students to learn.

'I think I got my love for Occupational Therapy from my dad and his love of the land and love of people and socialising.

Our house is a real 'ceili' house* and to me that's real OT and that's the type of OT that I would like to see continue.'

**"To call on a ceili' is a phrase used in Ireland meaning to call to the home of family or neighbours for a sociable visit. A 'Ceili house' is a house which was often full of visitors with lively story-telling and laughter.*

Thinking on your feet is so important. Children are unpredictable, all patients can be unpredictable, you have your risk assessment printed out, but you need to be alert and ready for the unexpected. Those skills are better learned by bringing students out and exploring real-life scenarios.

What attracted you to OT?

I came across it by chance, but what I like about OT is that we work across physical and mental health. We're holistic practitioners and I think what's unique about OT is that we can support somebody with their physical health and understand the impact this has on the mental health and vice versa. I am a real people person and I understand the impact of loneliness, isolation and grief and how detrimental that can be to your health, including your physical health. My OT career has changed and developed with me as my life and interests have matured. When I started initially, my interest was in mental health and learning disability. As I had my own four children, my interest in paediatrics grew, as did my interest in vocational rehabilitation. In a few years I might look at training in a different area - I like to keep learning new things and OT allows me to do that. I'm learning all the time.

'Becoming an OT was one of the best decisions I ever made.'

How would you like to see OT in the changing world of healthcare? Where do you see we could have a greater impact?

It depends when you ask me this question as every month it might change. But at the minute I would say we need to be more involved with education and within schools.

I would like to see a development of universal interventions where we would work with teachers, classroom assistants and parents to provide them with simple tips, tools and strategies that could be used within the classroom to build up those core skills, physical skills or mental health and well-being, looking at the person as an holistic being. Today in Northern Ireland there are commonly three-year waiting lists for Paediatric Occupational Therapy. I think if we can use the skills that we have, provide education to the service providers, whether that be in education, local community groups or voluntary organisations, then it might lessen the need for more specialist or targeted intervention.

You're doing this at the minute on a smaller scale?

Yes, my husband built an outdoor classroom for our local primary school and that's what we use every week. Many children don't have an awareness of emotions so we use simple strategies. Last week, we gave the children feathers and did breathing techniques with them. They came back the following week, and they were providing examples of how they used their feathers through the week. We bring in the horse and I demonstrate to them how he shows us when he is sad or happy. It is just something simple, but it's effective and the teachers can carry on these activities in the class. I would like to see more outdoor learning and outdoor classrooms.

Can you tell me about one time where you felt you really made a difference?

I have a great story about one child, her name is Ruby and I have permission to talk about her. She could talk about herself - she's brilliant, amazing! She could teach us all. She has quadriplegic cerebral palsy and a tracheostomy. When she came to us initially, she was not able to sit up without maximum support. I used a video to track her progress each week. Ruby had hippotherapy every week and with my husband carrying around her oxygen tank, she developed a very strong bond with her horse, Smokey. She was a very determined child and as the weeks went on, she progressed.

One day I looked at her and thought 'I think she might be able to weight bear,' so I put a gait belt on her and she could bear weight - it was amazing! We then got her to groom the horse as she was weight bearing so we could practice her standing. Then one day, she whispered, 'Walk?' She wanted to walk the pony! I gave her the rope and she took a few easy steps, and then the next week she was able to take more steps. After some practice she was able to lead that pony around the barn with limited assistance from us. Then, she was able to push the wheelbarrow around to tidy up after the horses. Her main goal was to attend mainstream school with her three older sisters, and she did that. That was a major accomplishment for her but also for my whole family. I couldn't have done it without the support of my family. It was nice for us all to be able to help someone in that way.

It never ceases to amaze me the impact that equine movement can have, but also the power of motivation. When Darragh spoke for the first time during his therapy his mother asked 'Why? How did that happen?' I couldn't really answer at that time because I was mesmerised. I was looking up all the research for answers but it always brings me back to motivation. He is in a real-life environment, not in a therapy room, there's natural lighting, he's not overstimulated. He was just enjoying that time with the horse like any other child.

> **'You know, you're doing a great job as an OT when you're not having to be there all the time, you have trained the person how to grade their own movement and how to get maximum benefit from the activity.**

I have learned especially from the farm that you don't have to be go, go, go all the time. Some of the best things happen when you let nature take over and you are there just to support.'

Can you sum up the Power of OT?

I would say it's the therapeutic use of self. I really see OT as a vocation. It doesn't feel like working. I feel I was born to be an Occupational Therapist. The Power of OT is the ability to use ourselves for the good of all our people, to help and support them. That's where I get my job satisfaction.

Martina's Key Takeaway: Nature can soothe, invigorate and heal a person, you don't always need expensive intervention, some of the best outcomes can be achieved from the natural environment.

14

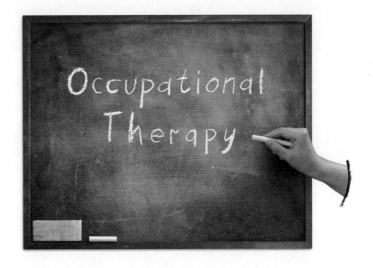

From Clinician
to Educator

In conversation with...

Anna O'Loughlin

Occupational Therapist, NHS
Lecturer, Ulster University

Northern Ireland

'My mum is a great role model - a wonderful person. She is of that generation of people who did not have the opportunities we now have, who are very resourceful, gifted with a range of living skills which they use to the full and are never idle.'

After 24 years in clinical practice gaining a wide range of experience in both the NHS and private sector, Anna recently made a career shift by taking up a post with Ulster University as a lecturer in Occupational Therapy.

Having clinical expertise is a major advantage for the students to prepare them for the world of work. We had an interesting conversation around Anna's hopes to enthuse, support and inspire the next generation of Occupational Therapists by preparing students as they make their journey from student to competent, confident and inspired clinician.

How did you become interested in healthcare and why OT?

A tragic event struck my aunt Sarah the year I was born which left her quadriplegic and dependent. She was a nurse in Dublin at the time and following her failed surgery she spent a year in the National Rehabilitation Centre in Dún Laoghaire before being transferred to what was the Route Hospital in Ballymoney, 30 minutes from our home. In the 1970s there was limited access to care facilities, specialist equipment and therapy services and as a result Sarah was a patient in Ballymoney for many years. Growing up we had the privilege of her company, laughter and love. Sarah became a central figure in the life of our family and without a second thought, my mum and dad brought her home every weekend and at school holiday times.

Learning to care for Sarah was natural and, in many ways, as children, we became her therapists - carrying out a range of activities with her which included passive movements of her joints, engaging her in social activities, reading, spelling, and quizzes as well as the basic tasks of feeding and personal care.

Unfortunately, the life lessons from Sarah did not immediately transfer into the 'A' Level grades necessary for me to enter straight into university. Looking for options, I attended an open day in Ulster University where I met Margaret, the course director for OT and was delighted to get a glimpse of a career I had never heard of.

Margaret was a very caring and motherly figure to me, very down to earth and could have held an audience regardless of who they were, such was her passion for OT. My own experience of caring for Sarah coupled with her talk that day, left me with the feeling that I was in the right place. I got to speak with Margaret and on leaving the room she had convinced me to repeat my 'A' Levels and come back to study OT.

What did you do before lecturing in Ulster University?

As an OT, I never considered myself a specialist, rather as an all-round generalist given my clinical experience. I started out as a Community OT before taking up a rotational post at the Ulster Hospital in Dundonald. I had only ever planned to stay for a year, but it was to become 17 great years. Initially, I felt I was too young to settle in one clinical area and too inexperienced to see my practice as holistic. I worked across every medical speciality within physical services at The Ulster and loved the variety and scope of OT within each one; however, my real passion lay in stroke rehabilitation and that is where I spent most of my career working within acute and sub-acute rehabilitation.

Following a move from The Ulster in later years, I enjoyed working in neurology and with rheumatology outpatients. I would advise any new graduate not to confine themselves to a single area of OT initially and to explore other areas of practice to build their knowledge and skills base. Having a breadth of knowledge and skills enabled me to have the confidence to work in private practice part-time, in addition to NHS practice. I have been working for The OT Practice since 2012 – the largest independent OT practice in the UK. Working for a company such as this is a great way to gain experience in the private sector and it offers great opportunities, welcome challenges and job satisfaction.

What personal characteristics do you bring to your professional role as an OT?

Caring for Sarah taught me core values of respect, humility, dignity, gratitude, patience, compassion and kindness - values I carry into every patient interaction.

One of my strengths as a clinician is my ability to develop rapport. The ability to recognise a person's situation and circumstances after a life-changing event such as stroke, or to recognise someone's pain or inability to do the simple tasks they used to do is so important. Putting the needs of the individual first, to listen deeply and understand them fully before the needs of the service is vital. Taking that one-to-one time with the patient is more important than getting them onto a wheelchair and going to the rehabilitation unit to get them involved with activity. Those first encounters are so important, the progress comes when the rapport is established. The patient must know, first and foremost, that we care and that we want to do what's best for them and with them.

I remember one patient reflecting on her stay within the stroke unit who told me that my ability to listen and to provide reassurance was more important to her than all the medical and nursing care she received.

Similarly, I recall a gentleman on the stroke unit with expressive aphasia who struggled to communicate his needs effectively. I took heart from how his shoulders dropped and how he relaxed when he saw me walk onto the ward. It was as if he was saying, 'Help is here. I'm going to be ok now.' The ability to recognise a patient's needs through body language is crucial.

Taking time with new patients and allowing them to have a voice in their treatment lays the foundations for a great working relationship. As clinicians, people's worries and anxieties are important considerations in our practice as we start to help them rebuild their life. This is an important skill and insight I bring to the university and to the students. It is not all about going straight in to do your assessment. How any situation feels to an individual is not any less important than how it looks.

Who has had the greatest impact overall in your role as a health care professional?

My mum is a great role model - a wonderful person. She is of that generation of people who did not have the opportunities we now have, who are very resourceful, gifted with a range of living skills which they use to the full and are never idle. I view her as a great example of how engagement in occupations has helped and continues to maintain her overall health and wellbeing. Many of the crafts and activities within Occupational Therapy which previously people would have considered less important, are now very much in vogue especially after the experience of lockdowns during COVID-19. People value and see the benefit in engaging in meaningful, purposeful occupations. Hopefully I can pass the baton to my children and others within my community to realise the value of 'doing.' My children and I are part of our local community garden and without realising it herself, my nine-year-old daughter is gaining positive mental health from this and as she says, 'It's hard to frown when you're out in the garden.'

My mum has influenced my ability to advocate for others, to ask questions, to find solutions, to be creative and to think outside the box. Certainly, as we worked with my aunt Sarah, we were always pushing the boundaries to find solutions to make her life as comfortable as possible. An example of this was the creation of a mechanical head support for Sarah who had lost the ability to lift her head off her chest due to years of poor postural management. Her flexed head position created skin breakdown under her chin and on her chest, causing pain. She lacked the ability to see and interact with her environment with reduced clarity of speech and reduced swallow.

We discussed and trialled different things to help but it was my brother's design of a motorised head unit for her wheelchair which helped her compensate for difficulties in a variety of areas. This device could be set on a cycle of motions which facilitated speaking and eating, for example. I remember the first time we used it at home, Sarah could identify what was on the TV, she could speak more clearly, eat and swallow better requiring only the assistance from one person, and it helped relieve the pressure on her skin.

What has helped you make the transition from clinician to educator?

Throughout my career I always had an underlying curiosity, and I have been driven to provide evidence-based practice and quality care to those in need by engaging in professional reading, attending courses to increase my skills and taking on new study. I enjoyed sharing new ideas and learning from others, and putting this into practice gave me great satisfaction. In clinical practice I was fortunate to be part of a progressive stroke team who were leading in the development and transformation of stroke services in our area and who were very research active. This prompted me to undertake a Master's degree in Stroke Practice which helped me explore my practice and it opened opportunities to become more involved in research activities. Now that I am in education, I hope to have the space and time to think about research and get involved in different areas of practice or education.

I have just completed a two-year postgraduate certificate in higher education practice which has given me a foundation and the tools to develop my skills as an effective educator. This transition from clinician to educator has been challenging and even daunting at a time when the programme for OT has been relocated across the country to a new campus but I am so excited about the journey ahead and the opportunity for new learning.

What do you hope for your students?

As a student I remember finding it difficult to fully grasp and define Occupational Therapy. Our unique skill of being able to reason and apply the understanding of occupation and its impact on health and wellbeing is often not as prominent as it should be.

Many challenges exist in clinical practice and there are well-publicised demands on healthcare resources which can maybe leave graduates feeling overwhelmed or daunted at the thought of a career in healthcare.

I want to use my clinical experience to empower students to be confident, assertive and courageous practitioners and to lead our profession effectively in the years ahead.

I hope to help students feel the sense of reward and joy from their interactions with and for people who experience difficulties with their activities of daily living. I am encouraged by some of the conversations I have had with students during their practice-based learning, and I am heartened to see their growth, enthusiasm, confidence, sensitivity, and initiative develop. I love to see students being proactive - going the extra mile and putting themselves forward so that they gain as much as possible from their experiences. I hope that I can influence and educate students to be the type of colleague that I would enjoy working with in a clinical setting.

Where do you see Power of OT?

One can only imagine how many different aspects of aunt Sarah's life could have been improved if the field of OT then had been as developed as it is now. The Power of OT lies in our ability to place the people at the centre of our interventions and use our holistic approach to improve and overcome the challenges which they face.

Martina's Key Takeaway: Being a strong role model is the most powerful form of educating.

"Rest and self-care are so important.
When you take time to replenish
your spirit, it allows you to
serve others from the overflow.
You cannot serve from an empty vessel."

Eleanor Brownn

15

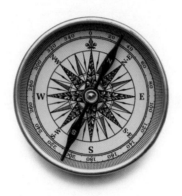

Navigating Through Unexpected Crisis

Mairia Mulholland

Occupational Therapist
Mental Health & Paediatrics

Northern Ireland

'One of the most impactful parts of our
learning in university was when we had
opportunities to speak to service users who
came to the university and talked about
their personal experience of disability.
I will never forget the stories they told and
how it made me feel when hearing how
OT intervention helped them.'

Mairia is just three years post-qualification and was one of the cohorts of OT students who trained during the COVID-19 pandemic. Having heard from Course Lecturers, Clare McMonagle and Anna O'Loughlin, I felt it was important to also include the thoughts of a recently qualified OT on her training, the clinical placements, making the transition from student to clinician and finding her feet in the workplace.

How did you initially find out about Occupational Therapy?

I first discovered Occupational Therapy through my careers advisor in school. While I was looking for work experience aged 16, the teacher connected me with an Occupational Therapist who worked in mental health. I spent a day visiting the OT department that I later ended up working in post-qualifying. Even though I had known I wanted to work in healthcare, I had never heard about OT before this visit. From that first encounter, I loved it. My previous experiences with hospitals had always felt somewhat morbid and illness-focused, but OT was so much more about the person. Soon after this, I attended an open day at Ulster University where I got a better understanding of the role, and it further reinforced my decision to pursue a career in OT.

How did you enjoy the university course?

As with most university courses, there are parts of the OT course which are more beneficial than others. Certain elements and modules of the course help new graduates hit the ground running once you enter the professional world. Many of our lecturers were experienced professionals and conversations with them contributed significantly to understanding the unique demands of the different services and areas of practice. Although the theory and the knowledge are instrumental in developing student confidence, I felt that I only truly began to understand the role and the importance of OT when I was seeing it day-to-day during my practice placements. Throughout the course, I had four practice placements and one role-emerging placement. Placements are a great tool in allowing students to gain comprehensive experience in different areas of OT practice and the university did their best to ensure students had the opportunity to gain experience in a range of areas. I think the variety of placements are crucial in figuring out which area could suit you best. Although placements give you great real-world experience of what it is like in the day-to-day world of OT, I feel that it's not until you are really immersed in the field after qualifying that you can decide what really works best for you. I also think it's vital for newly qualified OTs to try different areas of work before settling on a permanent one.

One of the most impactful parts of our learning in university was when we had opportunities to speak to service users who came to the university and talked about their personal experience of disability. I will never forget the stories they told and how it made me feel when hearing how OT intervention helped them. Overall, I think the range of learning from the university, but more importantly the clinical experience from placements provided a good grounding for employment.

It may sound obvious but to help apply for jobs after graduation, I would recommend that at the very beginning of their course, OT students research the required experience and job skills and keep a record of their key experiences starting with the very first placement. It's surprising how easily you can forget these things when it comes to applying for jobs even as little as three years later!

You were a student during COVID-19. Did that have an impact on navigating placements or what you were able to learn from them?

We were lucky that the university had some flexibility in arranging placements to ensure we were gaining as much experience as possible throughout the three years. For instance, I didn't initially have a placement in an acute setting, but I managed to get it changed by contacting the relevant department and putting forward my reasons for requesting a change. The COVID-19 pandemic did have a significant impact and it certainly was challenging, but in hindsight, it was probably beneficial because as OTs, we are natural problem-solvers and this only helped me develop these skills further as well as providing experience navigating through unexpected crisis. As undergraduates without much experience, we had to find innovative ways to deliver care whilst ensuring everyone's safety - this provided a unique but valuable learning opportunity although didn't come without its challenges.

One of my placements during the pandemic involved working in a respiratory ward where the staff were under immense pressure to free up much-needed hospital beds. Patients recovering from COVID-19 and suffering from long COVID faced significant challenges, such as losing their physical strength and skills after prolonged ICU stays. Carrying out functional assessments and intervention programmes was very difficult. This experience highlighted the importance of adaptive problem-solving and flexibility in care delivery.

My role-emerging placement was in a residential refuge for women and children who were affected by domestic abuse. The purpose of a role-emerging placement was to go into a service which currently had no OT input and try to implement an OT programme within it. We had planned various mental health groupwork and self-care activities, but at short notice new pandemic restrictions meant the residents had to isolate in their rooms, preventing any group interactions. This situation required creative thinking to deliver care effectively under the constraints.

During my placements, managing stress was crucial. We had designated placement coordinators who were available to offer support as we needed it. I also found that when I began working, Senior OTs were more than happy to lend a listening ear and offer advice. I often find that if I'm feeling stressed about an issue in work, discussing it with experienced OTs or OT Assistants can often make it feel much more manageable, even if it's only a five-minute chat over a coffee.

After finishing university, how did you choose a speciality, did you know which area you wanted to work in?

After graduating, I was drawn towards working in mental health having seen real patient improvements during my placements. I believe you need a particular kind of personality to work in mental health and I thought it suited mine. It felt right for me as I like to think I am easy-going and try to have a calm, relaxed energy when things don't go to plan. I have patience, which is crucial when working in mental health as progress can be slow at times and there can be many setbacks along the way.

'As mental health OTs, we are prepared to measure progress very slowly, we accept there may not be huge wins every day, but to celebrate all the small wins which is so important for the client.'

Can you tell me about your first job in mental health and the role of an OT in that setting?

My first job was in a mental health hospital. I worked with both inpatients and outpatients. For outpatients, the goal was to help them regain confidence and reintegrate into the community. This was achieved by them participating in sporting or leisure activities or seemingly basic tasks like grocery shopping or visiting a coffee shop. The focus was on tailoring the goals to the individual's needs, helping them gain independence and overcome their fears or limitations. As with most OT services, it was very patient focused, so we collaboratively discussed with the client what was important to them and what they needed to achieve to live as independently as possible.

Working with inpatients involved a similar process of setting personalised goals, but the progress was often slower due to the instability of their mental health and the complexity of their conditions. The aim was to help them achieve functional improvements at their own pace, recognising that their mental state and therefore abilities could fluctuate significantly from day to day.

As an OT working in mental health, we really try to focus on the positives and what the individual can do. Due to the nature of some mental illnesses and through no fault of their own, service users at times can find it difficult to focus in on these positives. That is why it was always important as an OT in mental health to really emphasise that the small wins are often actually big and important wins for these individuals.

How do you personally decompress after a stressful day?

A great thing about working in mental health is that I can use the exact same techniques I encourage my patients to use and I have a heightened awareness about when I might need to implement them for myself. I find that relaxation, finding an activity that interests me, talking to others, a good laugh and even something as simple as getting out and getting some fresh air all work wonders for me.

I tend to be a chatterbox so if there are issues with a client or something on my mind, I discuss it with a colleague. Often, I realise after talking it through, that the problem is nowhere near as big as it may have seemed.

You've recently transitioned to a new role in Paediatrics and Learning Disabilities (LD), what made you make the change?

My transition to working with Paediatrics and LD was partly driven by a desire for career growth and personal development. Whilst I enjoyed my time in mental health and learned a lot from it, I felt the need to explore other areas of OT. I believe it's important to gain a broad range of experiences before settling into a specific niche. Although it has only been a few months, working in Paediatrics and LD has offered a new set of challenges and learning opportunities and is already further enhancing my skills as an OT.

How do you feel that OT fits into a multidisciplinary team?

In my career so far, I have noticed that OT often requires advocating for the profession's value and the impact it has on patients' lives. While other healthcare roles might have more immediately visible outcomes, the changes brought about by OT can be more subtle but are equally significant and arguably longer lasting. It may not be as measurable as nursing or a medical intervention, but we must advocate for the work we do.

I have really enjoyed working within multidisciplinary teams, such as with psychiatrists, psychologists, social workers, and nurses, and this has been instrumental in providing comprehensive patient care. Thankfully as an OT, I have never felt undervalued or overlooked in any team I have been part of. That said, I do think it's important that we continue to highlight the unique contributions that OT can bring to the MDT and even to those in our personal lives. I often have friends and family joke that I spend my days going out for coffee or going shopping, not realising that what we are doing is supporting someone in getting elements of their independence back that they may have been struggling with for years.

What is your ambition for the future?

Looking to the future, I hope to continue exploring different areas within OT to find what I enjoy the most. I aim to maintain my enthusiasm for the job and avoid feeling stagnant. The breadth of OT allows for continuous learning and development, which keeps the profession exciting and fulfilling. Additionally, understanding the holistic impact of mental and physical health on a person's overall well-being is crucial, and I strive to incorporate this perspective in all my work.

What do you see is the Power of OT?

Whether in physical or mental health, the value and Power of Occupational Therapy lies in our focus on the person rather than the illness. It emphasises the positives and capabilities of individuals as opposed to the limitations caused by their illness. Celebrating small wins with clients, encourages me to do the same in my own life. This approach not only makes the job rewarding but also significantly improves the quality of life of the people we serve.

Martina's Key Takeaway: Celebrating small achievements is an important way to track incremental progress and it makes the person feel good more often.

16

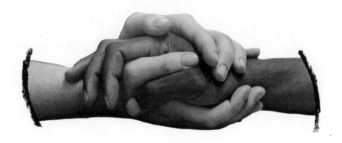

Dignity, Kindness
and Compassion

Norma Jane Findlay

Occupational Therapist & Clinical Director
Training for Care

Scotland

'For anyone who has community experience, especially in working with those who have very complex needs and understands how an injury can impact their ability to function in life, I would encourage them to consider legal work because if we don't have more OTs in this field, then we don't have that holistic picture.'

I first met Norma in Edinburgh when I spoke at the Conference for the RCOTSS-IP (Royal College of Occupational Therapy Specialist Section for Independent Practice.) She had been familiar with Seating Matters for many years due to her interest in the importance of considering 24-hour postural care. It was clear from our first meeting that she was passionate and dedicated to her profession and patients. Her knowledge and enthusiasm were infectious, and I felt good after spending time with her. She then read my autobiography and was very keen to visit the Seating Matters factory and learn more about manufacturing and the processes involved in building a therapeutic chair. It was evident from the start that we had a lot in common, not least our passion for Occupational Therapy. When she visited me at the factory, we had the following conversation which I found really uplifting.

What's your current role?

My current role is a clinical director within an expert witness company. I train and supervise Occupational Therapists, Physiotherapists and Nurses. We prepare reports for the courts providing details of the many care needs people may have following catastrophic injury, brain injury or amputation and we also cover clinical negligence cases. It's a very holistic assessment of all their needs.

When we assess someone's care needs, we need to quantify those in terms of their daily routine. So, we look at that from the moment the person gets up in the morning, all through the day and night. It's a 24-hour picture of what their needs are. It's not just their care needs, it's their equipment needs, their adaptation needs, accommodation needs, holiday needs etc. So, in its fullest, it's what provides quality of life. As an Occupational Therapist, we are trained to look at how the person can maximise their independence and their quality of life, so our skills fit in very well with the role of the expert witness.

When we consider support for a catastrophic accident, we say 'but for" the accident what would their life have looked like?' We make recommendations so they can reach the fullest potential that their life would have been before the accident. That also applies if it was a birth injury. So, for example, in cerebral palsy, we look at how that child would have functioned within their family, what their daily routine would have looked like 'but for' the accident. We will make our recommendations which often overlaps with their physical therapy and speech and language therapy needs.

Is this an area of Occupational Therapy which you would encourage other OTs to consider and if so, why?

Yes, I would. As Occupational Therapists, we have an important role to inform the courts. As a Community Occupational Therapist with over 20 years' experience, I often worked with those who had been involved in injury where litigation was involved. We work with the instructing solicitors to gain access to all the equipment and therapies the person needs. We need to ensure that the report is comprehensive and that takes a highly experienced, qualified Occupational Therapist. So, for anyone who has community experience, especially in working with those who have very complex needs and understands how an injury can impact their ability to function in life, I would encourage them to consider legal work because if we don't have more Occupational Therapists becoming carer experts*, then we don't have that holistic picture. Being able to provide a good report to the court is the only way we can truly meet the needs of the person. It's so important at that time to get it right, you may only have that one chance of doing so.

I have seen that whilst there are certain conditions with which you wouldn't usually anticipate improvement, we do see that if the correct therapy or equipment is provided then secondary complications and destructive postures can be avoided. For example, as Occupational Therapists, we need to ensure that we provide all of the necessary recommendations to prevent any further deterioration. If we fail to do that within the report, then there are no allowances made for ongoing support. I feel it's important that anyone becoming a carer expert should have a minimum of seven years post-qualification experience and ideally having a very good understanding of how individuals live within their home settings and in the community.

You are also the Manual Handling Course Director at Training for Care. How did you become interested in this area of OT?

Training for Care is an educational charity where we specialise in social care and childcare training. My interest in postural care, moving and assisting goes back to when I was just newly qualified. I was quite clear that I wanted to work with those with complex needs. I started in two centres for adults with neurological impairment. What I was observing was people with a disability were being moved from A to B, but not often in a way that I

* *Carer expert is used here to mean an expert legal witness.*

would describe as with dignity, kindness and compassion. That's not a judgment on the people who were supporting their move, it's just that they hadn't been given correct guidance, training and information. Interestingly, that task fell to me, that was part of my job. So, I needed to make sure that if I was responsible for everyone within the service being moved and positioned in a way which was with kindness, care and compassion, using hoists and slings, etc. I realised that I needed to upskill myself within that area and so that's what I did.

After realising the importance of moving and assisting and positioning, realising the importance for function and how that impacted on occupation, I then attended other courses to upskill. I began to question whether what we were doing really did encompass that full occupation and positioning as well as moving and assisting, incorporating safe use of hoist as well as considering posture. So, I decided to take on the role of trainer around 2009 and a while later I took on the role of Director of Training and began to drive home a really person-centred approach.

It's not just teaching about regulations in using hoists or other equipment. It's about moving someone in a way that respects the individual and really appreciates that from the moment you wake up in the morning if you need to have this kind of assistance, that it is provided in such a way that recognises the importance of kindness of touch. We hope that by training people well in these areas that we are contributing to improving care standards.

What attracted you to the OT profession?

I always knew I would work in a healthcare profession but not necessarily OT. My auntie, who isn't too much older than me, has cerebral palsy and as a child I grew up aware of her needs. She had significant support requirements and needed to have all care provided for her. Then as I got into teenage years, I became much more appreciative of the extent of those care needs. She had to be cared for by paid carers eventually, when other family passed away. I saw examples of good care and not so good care and I began to recognise the importance of good care. For me, providing good care and really enhancing quality of life was key. I remember being introduced to Physiotherapy. I could see the importance of a gym and exercise, etc., but it didn't quite resonate entirely with me. Then I was introduced to Community OT, and I could really see how that would make a difference. I chose to specialise in Occupational Therapy. So now I've taken on, I wouldn't say 'responsibility' because it's a pleasure that I have, the role of welfare guardian for my auntie. I make sure that she has access to the slings, hoists, chairs and everything that she needs so it's great for her care. It's interesting being on the other side as a guardian and as a relative working with her Occupational Therapists and the care staff.

There was one occasion where my auntie was assessed for a specialised chair, but the local authority would not provide it, and whilst I could have purchased it privately, I felt that by doing so I was not reflecting the needs of everyone else who needed specialised seating. I felt I needed to demonstrate to the local authority that this was not just a chair for comfort it was for protecting body shape, reducing secondary complications and improving function. I had done a lot of research in this area and because of this the local authority agreed to purchase the chair and now they provide bespoke chairs for those with complex disabilities.

In your role as an OT have there been any role models or people who inspired you?

When I worked within the neurological services, I had the true pleasure of being mentored and supervised by an OT called Linda Gibson. She was also my anatomy and physiology lecturer at university and had taught in Hong Kong for many years working with people with neurological impairment. I was encouraged and I learned from the best in the early days so I could really see how she applied Occupational Therapy to everyday life. Rather than seeing a patient as someone who has experienced a stroke who we need to do ten repetitions of extension and flexion every day, we're going to think about their interests, what's important to them and then use meaningful activity to get the person's cooperation and ultimately improve their function. It was important to have that early on in my career to let me see the valuable skills of Occupational Therapists. I still don't think as a profession we have embraced our true value.

Tell me about the vocational rehabilitation service you set up?

Through the medical legal work, we had clients who were unable to return to work post injury and I knew this was a specialism within Occupational Therapy. But it wasn't my specialism, and I couldn't guarantee that the Occupational Therapist recommendations that I was making would fully meet those needs. A large proportion of the people that I would assess post-injury had a career which they loved but were unable to return to work. So now we've created a service where Occupational Therapists deliver vocational rehabilitation, and we can refer for that. It was an area of unmet need, and one which OTs can excel in. We need to be looking at the person's full picture again, because whilst some reports may say the person is unable to return to work, they might be unable to return to their previous employment or their career. But as human beings, we need to do something, we need to look at alternative employment or activity. For example, there could be an individual with an acquired brain injury who might be looking at voluntary positions part-time. They need an experienced OT with vocational expertise who can assess and advise and work with the person, so they are getting the most out of life post-injury.

Where would you like to see more development in Occupational Therapy?

I would like to see more attention and training on 24-hour postural care, moving and assisting and not just for those who have complex needs. It starts with anyone who has limited mobility where we notice body shape changes. Occupational Therapists play a key role in that. The moment that you start to see a reduction in mobility, Occupational Therapists are often asked to come in assess for falls or bath transfers. But in my mind, we need to look at how the person is sitting, lying, standing and walking. We need to be concerned with 24-hour postural care and position as that is really key to how a person functions and how we maximise their independence. We need to prevent any deterioration in their body shape to be able to maximise function.

Going back to what ignited my interest in Occupational Therapy in the first place, the personal experience with my auntie, often if someone has either cerebral palsy or any neurological impairment or indeed any disability, there's an assumption that their body shape will change, almost like an expectation that they will have secondary complications. In my experience, we need to challenge that and put effort into preventing secondary complications and those destructive postures. I think Occupational Therapists are best placed to help the individual avoid the secondary complications and provide the care that they need.

'We need to challenge the assumption that secondary complications and destructive postures are an inevitable consequence for people with complex disabilities.'

Posture influences not just pressure care but also swallowing, respiration, digestion, bladder and bowel function so we need to be more aware of the benefits of 24-hour postural positioning in protecting body shape and reducing secondary complications.

What is the Power of OT?

I think the Power of Occupational Therapy is working with people to fulfil their potential and to live a life which is enjoyable, joyful, purposeful, and allows them to engage in all the activities they would want to participate in. As Occupational Therapists, we can ascertain what those wishes and dreams are and assist them to fulfil their potential. In the work I do even the process of taking the time to sit with someone and listen, is seen as a real benefit for some people. Giving them the time to sit down and talk through what they want to achieve in the future we hope that by the end of the process our recommendations will have helped them fulfil their goals and aspirations.

I find the community of Occupational Therapy extremely important and valuable, and it really makes the profession worthwhile. Our community is amazing. If we go to a conference and meet with colleagues, there's just an understanding that we have the best interests of those that we work with at heart. I will do everything I can to assist you with what you need to achieve and vice versa. Our purpose is around helping each other and that involves sharing our learning and new ideas.

Martina's Key Takeaway: Compassion is usefully described as a sensitivity to distress, together with the commitment, courage and wisdom to do something about it. There is evidence that compassionate relationships have significant physiological effects, for instance influencing heart rates, breathing and other internal systems, including our brains (Cole-King & Gilbert, 2011.) As OTs we need to take the time to show compassion to our patients, families and carers.

17

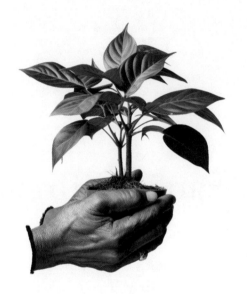

The Blue Zone

Paraig O'Brien

Fellow of the RCOT
Retired Occupational Therapist Manager, NHS

Northern Ireland

'I strongly believe purposeful, satisfying activity is right at the heart of the whole profession.'

I first met Paraig when I worked as a Community Occupational Therapist in Foyle NHS health trust in Northern Ireland. He was the Head OT Manager responsible for community services. His dedication to the staff, the clients, and the community as well as his profession was outstanding. I would give Paraig full credit and recognition for the development of the OT service in the Foyle health trust area. He recognised the unmet needs of the community, and he was confident and enthusiastic that a fully operational OT service was vital in meeting those needs. He saw there was inequality for the community in the Northwest area of Northern Ireland and set about changing that. He was committed to developing the credibility of the OT service along with improving the services for the community. During his 10 years in that post, he was responsible for creating 36 new OT posts in the community, paediatrics, and support staff.

When I first started this project, he was one of the first OTs to come to mind to invite for interview. He has been very influential in advocating for Occupational Therapy and his contribution to education, research, legislation, and policy changes particularly in housing standards, has been widely recognised by his peers across the UK and further afield. I am delighted that he agreed to contribute to 'The Power of OT.'

Your resumé is very long and interesting, why did you choose OT?

I was attracted to OT because I was fascinated by both the arts and the sciences in equal measure. My mother taught me to play violin from a young age, I wanted to go to art college and had a particular interest in architecture and product design, but I also loved the science world of physics and biology too. So, I wondered how I could combine all these interests and I saw that OT had that potential. It combines the arts and sciences well and can attract people with quite diverse interests. My aunt Brenda was an OT, the first in the family, and I talked to her about the profession. She had trained in Astley Ainsley in Scotland as there was no OT training course in Northern Ireland at the time.

It was during a visit with a Community OT working on housing issues in Ballymena that helped me develop a special interest in community care and made me think, 'I want to do this job.' It was so practical; you could see the difference it made in people's lives right away.

So, thanks to my aunt Brenda and that Community OT called Eileen, I made my decision to apply. Interestingly, my daughter Orla is the latest generation in our family to join the OT profession where she combines Occupational Therapy with a range of complementary therapies.

Tell me about your first job and the impact the Northern Irish Troubles* had on your career.

Straight after qualifying in the early 1980s, I went to work as a Community OT in the Belfast conflict areas of 'The Shankill' and 'The Falls.' It was a particularly violent time in Northern Ireland. Reflecting on how the conflict affected our work, we planned our visits by the columns of smoke rising on the horizon! I can remember saying 'I can't see Mrs Murphy today due to the rioting

---

*The Troubles is the name given to the period of civil war in Northern Ireland between the 1970s and 1990s where many lives were lost on both sides of the conflict.

in her area; Must try to get to her tomorrow.'

Several times people tried to hijack my car and burn it. At one stage they put timber and other combustibles around it, it was about to go up in flames when I retrieved it. Other times I had to drive round burning barricades, avoiding guys with balaclavas (ski masks) to get OTs out on home visits.

It was easy for uninvolved people to get caught in the middle of a conflict situation, particularly when you had to work there and couldn't avoid an area. There were times we were caught up in crossfire from gun fights or in the middle of plastic bullet and rioting exchanges. I worked with several people permanently disabled by plastic bullets when working in Neurorehab in the Royal Hospital and then nearly got hit by one myself going out for a sandwich at lunchtime one day.

What sort of support or counselling was available to staff at that time?

There was no formal counselling really but we had an exceptionally good Head of Service who had great knowledge, skill and compassion.

There was one day where I got shot in the neck when I was simply lifting bathing equipment out of the back of the car. I felt a stinging sensation in the left side of my neck and blood started to run down my neck. I thought I had been stung by a bee but I went to see a welfare officer nearby and he said 'You have been shot!'

That had an impact on me in terms of my work. I asked my manager if it was ok if I didn't go into that area again until I got over it. But I went back after a couple of weeks, we all just got on with the job.

In 1998 the worst bombing in Northern Ireland occurred in a town called Omagh leading to 29 deaths and over 200 wounded, many permanently both physically and in terms of mental health. It happened at a time when most people believed that the 30-year conflict was coming to an end.

I will never forget the vision of multiple funeral processions making their way along the roads as my colleague and I were travelling to Omagh to provide support in the days immediately after the bomb. We were tasked with the important role of emergency planning for the survivors, calculating how many wheelchairs, adaptations and dedicated OT staff would be needed to help in the aftermath.

There were also occasions where dedicated debriefing services were required for therapists. Although we got on with it, it did affect all our lives to varying degrees.

Even though the conflict is now officially 'over,' many thousands of people live with physical disabilities that will require ongoing support for the rest of their lives and many thousands more will need ongoing support with unresolved mental health issues.

On reflection there is much more that Occupational Therapists could and should share regarding their experiences of the impact Northern Irish conflict had on their lives and practice.

Many people reading this would never have considered how significant the role of the OT was during the conflict. Thank you for highlighting that and bringing it to the attention of others.

Can we now talk about another significant part of your career, product design?

When recommending equipment I observed that often it was poorly designed, resulting in significant non-use. I was one of the first OTs from Northern Ireland to seek a dual qualification in product design for disabled people and OT. I went to the London College of Furniture where I was part of an educational process that completely influenced the rest of my career. I realised that no one person has all the skills to meet the challenges of disability but with interprofessional collaboration you can get much better outcomes. At the London College of Furniture there were people from the technical world, product designers, architects, engineers and people from the life sciences. I was in the life science world with Speech and Language Therapists, Physiotherapists and Occupational Therapists. We set up interprofessional task groups to design products for disabled people. We learned about design and the manufacturing process, and they learned about disability. That model never left me, right through to the government work I did later; working collaboratively across professions and departments, harnessing expertise, focused on the needs and challenges of disability.

'I was grateful to receive the Demand Prize for the best Disability Design Research Dissertation.'

Following on from the postgraduate diploma in product design for disability, I was offered a very interesting research job in Oxford to set up clinical trials of disability equipment. We had to work at speed, six months maximum, to look at a product area, e.g., outdoor transport systems, all the new wheelchairs in the UK or home management products. My job was to set up clinical trials, undertake expert appraisals including health and safety checks, and get consumer feedback. I learned so much working again in collaboration with bioengineers and discovered the power of service user engagement to give you quality feedback. We provided feedback on our findings to the industry to let them know where to improve their products. It was free research and development for industry, service users felt empowered to have their voices heard and in shaping the future of product design, and therapists had better evidence-based data to choose assistive technologies.

In 2010 I received a Fellowship from the RCOT. It was a genuinely lovely experience. I was humbled by the sheer amount of time and energy colleagues put into making these submissions for fellowship awards - it is an onerous task. I am deeply indebted to colleagues and honoured to be recognised by my peers. I was also very pleased to receive 'The Inspirational Colleague Award,' which was organised by the Chartered Institute of Housing and delivered by the Housing Minister for the Department of Communities. I was incredibly grateful to have been recognised outside my own professional field. It was a formal recognition and positive affirmation of the success of collaborative cross-sector working.

Tell me about your role in changing legislation and policy for wheelchair housing.

I knew there was something fundamentally wrong with the design of wheelchair-standard housing. It had not been reviewed to meet the demands of modern community care. The previous standards did not look at the ergonomics of the assisted wheelchair user, carer and new moving and handling equipment that had come into place since the introduction of Manual Handling Operations Regulation (MHOR 1992.) It was assumed that the average wheelchair user was a self-propelling, independent user and space standards reflected that assumption. We now know from statistics that the average wheelchair user is assisted. Therefore, in applying inclusive design principles to suit everyone, we needed to increase space standards to accommodate assisted wheelchair users and their carers in new-build housing.

I set out to prove this through my Master's research programme. I undertook a critical review of the UK and Irish standards for wheelchair housing, looking at the underpinning ergonomics, anthropometry and other research studies. I also examined law and policy where I could see clear gaps. Since then, I have become even more convinced because I have looked at the scale of musculoskeletal injuries amongst carers which is significant, but I believe further work is needed in this area. Injuries to statutory carers are covered by RIDDOR* but for so

*RIDDOR *The Reporting of Injuries, Diseases and Dangerous Occurrences Regulations 2013 is a UK law that requires employers, and other people in charge of work premises, to report and keep records of work-related accidents, injuries and fatalities.*

many informal or family carers there is no strategic system to monitor musculoskeletal injury. People may be getting injured when moving and handling their loved ones and if the unpaid care had to be paid for at the same rate as statutory care, it would cost millions.

The Master's I completed conclusively proved that there needed to be a radical rethink of wheelchair housing standards.

> **'My research established that there needed to be a radical shift in the paradigm of wheelchair standard housing in the whole of the UK and Ireland. So I set out from that day to utilise research findings to change government policy and design standards for wheelchair standard housing. The journey was to take 17 years from 1999-2016.'**

At that time, I worked in Ulster University, first as a part-time lecturer and then full-time. I concentrated on community studies and commenced further research and publication into disability design. I was seconded from the university to help government with its first major review of housing adaptations in Northern Ireland. I had strong leadership offered by Nuala McArdle (OT) at the Department of Health and David Bass from the Northern Ireland Housing Executive* (NIHE,) who has sadly passed away since. Together they had a vision to create a new type of OT post, a Housing Adaptations Liaison Manager placed in a government setting. The role was to facilitate collaborative working between

Northern Ireland Housing Executive is the public housing authority for Northern Ireland and is responsible for the provision of social housing which meets the needs of citizens.

the Department of Health and the Northern Ireland Housing Executive at all levels and to initiate much needed change. It was a radical concept to select an Occupational Therapist to coordinate interdepartmental working at the highest level.

How did you find that role? Did you get cooperation and recognition?

It was fantastic! I never worried about OT not being recognised. I approached the role with the skills and ethos I had learned and used in London, identifying the problems disabled people have with the systems of housing adaptation delivery. We mapped it out with very strong service user engagement from the charity Disability Action.

We examined where the system was failing people in terms of an efficient, effective service and then we looked at the skillsets across all agencies: housing; health and procurement to see how they could shape a better delivery system.

We were not trying to specifically prove the worth of the OT but looked at the skillsets of every profession. We formed cross-professional task groups to look at the problem areas such as lifts, complex case management, design standards, communications and user engagement.

The task groups included all relevant stakeholders - policy makers, architects, designers, OTs and people with disabilities. By working together to solve problems for disabled people we all learned about each other's skills and roles. Wonderful respect built up between housing and health. Before that time there were some undercurrents and professional tensions, but this joint working with the authority of a government review made a difference. It really improved the understanding of the skills the OT brought to the table.

I had a keen user focus as I was continually interested in the challenges disabled people were facing. If I felt any professional was steering off course, I would say

'Let's bring focus back on the service user.'

The fact that I had dual training, Occupational Therapy with a Master's in environmental design and a postgraduate diploma in product design helped me to see challenges in terms of housing perspectives, including design and delivery processes.

How long were you in that post?

It was a two-year secondment from the university. I then returned to the university to complete my five-year contract.

Following that I went to work in Donegal and learned about working in the Republic of Ireland. They were two very happy years working with a great team in an idyllic, rural setting. It was so peaceful to work in a quiet, countryside area after working in highly pressurised urban settings. There was a cultural difference in the countryside. People were very independent and resilient, expressing deep gratitude for any help they received and there was a strong sense of community cohesion.

It was also a new model for the Republic of Ireland, placing OTs in primary care teams for the first time. I chose it because I wanted to influence this new model, I wanted to make a valuable contribution, so they would want to employ OTs in every primary care team in the Republic of Ireland. I achieved my objective after two years and there are now OTs routinely in primary care teams.

It was a very productive two years as I was working part-time in Donegal delivering HSE work whilst also undertaking consultancy work with the Housing Executive, carrying out an in-depth review of the needs of wheelchair users. I was building on the objective of the Master's, I wanted to strengthen the evidence base so that I could change policy and the way houses were being built.

The research was funded by the Northern Ireland Housing

Executive where I undertook thirty-one detailed research interviews with wheelchair users and their families about the design of their homes, element by element. We discussed the answers to some questions – 'What works well in your house? What does not work for you? How can the system be improved?'

I developed a new planning system for wheelchair users. When an OT assessed a person for a new wheelchair, anonymised data was transferred to housing planners to decide how many new wheelchair houses were needed in Northern Ireland, where to build them and to what standard.

A permanent Housing Adaptations Liaison Manager post was created which I then held for years. I contributed to the first interdepartmental review of Northern Ireland Housing Adaptations Services, but on the second time around I was coordinating the review. Having reviewed and developed the methodology during the first review, we expanded the scope to include new-build accessible housing and the creation of a register of accessible housing and adaptations. I realised that if you are constantly doing the same adaptations in older housing, we must design these missing elements into new-build housing as standard.

Northern Ireland was the first UK jurisdiction to adopt Lifetimes Homes for all its new social housing from 1998. I was involved in a major evaluation of costs and benefits of Lifetime Homes where we looked at the user benefits and the costs, to make the case for the Lifetime Homes concept, not just for Northern Ireland but also for other housing services across UK and Ireland. A house type that could meet the growing and changing needs of service users over their lifetimes. It might be to address the needs of young children and their parents, then as the people grow older and mobility changes, we need a house type which already has access features subtly built in, reducing the scale and the cost of adaptations or the pressure to move house later in life.

The emerging evidence base was widely distributed through UK anti-poverty social charity Joseph Rowntree Foundation, and the Chartered Institute of Housing. It is still often cited for other housing providers to consider this type of housing. In N. Ireland, 90% of new-build social housing is Lifetime Homes standard and 10% wheelchair standard. Our research helped to build the evidence base for these standards, and I believe they should also be considered for new-build private sector developments.

You have been very influential in developing policies and standards for housing adaptations and home environmental controls which have had a very positive impact for people living with disability. Can you share what you consider to be your greatest achievement?

One of the biggest achievements was the changes to legislation and policy regarding the Disabled Facility Grant (DFG) means-testing of families with disabled children. Through professional research, effective public campaigning, and a formal departmental review, means-testing for paediatric support was abolished in Northern Ireland in 2004.

Until that time many families with disabled children were forced to pull out of the grants system as they could not afford the adaptations which were required. OTs identified the undisputed need, but the families withdrew due to financial pressure. I needed to prove the scale and nature of this phenomena and wrote a research paper which was published by British Journal of Occupational Therapy (BJOT.) I approached the OT services in N. Ireland to find out how many families with genuine needs were pulling out of the system for financial or other reasons. There was quite conclusive evidence that there was a major problem.

We had a great service user campaigner, Brendan McKeever, who was working tirelessly to access a range of services for his disabled son. He realised that the issues he was experiencing, including the unfairness of the DFG means-testing, were being shared by many families around the UK.

Because of the job I was in at the time we had access to policymakers and decision-makers. We were starting to change government perception partly through OT research evidence, and partly through Brendan's campaigning. He was very good at harnessing engagement across broad sections of society and so achieved cross-party political support.

We managed to change the legislation in Northern Ireland and that was a profound experience. It meant that the income or resources of the families of the disabled child were no longer means-tested. This change, and increasing the upper threshold of DFG grant-aid, resulted in an incremental improvement in the delivery of much-needed adaptations for families of disabled children.

The essential problem with the means-testing methodology was that often the extra costs of disability were not factored in and family outgoings were not considered, just the incomes.

I can still remember the government announcement event, it was a truly wonderful experience which will always stay with me. Brendan was invited to attend a surprise presentation where it was formally announced that means-testing had been abolished. He was temporarily stunned into silence and then there was a huge cheer from the large gathering. It was a very emotional day for all of us, we enjoyed the sheer joy of this long, hard campaign coming to fruition. But it did not stop there. Frances Heywood, a colleague and wonderful mentor from Bristol University, was a researcher on housing and social policy in England. She had delivered many excellent publications on adaptations and housing became involved. She could see that if DFG means-testing could be abolished in Northern Ireland, it could also influence policy in the rest of the UK.

She and Brendan, in collaboration with the Joseph Rowntree Foundation, Contact-a-Family and other bodies used the model in Northern Ireland to lobby for a change in the law throughout the UK and they succeeded in Wales and then England. It very rarely happens that changes in Northern Ireland begin a chain reaction in other places. When the announcement was delivered in Westminster it was a truly memorable and exciting day.

As with so many OTs, even in retirement you can't quite seem to move away from the profession... For those who do not know your story can you give us an overview of this latest stage of your career?

Until recently, I undertook occasional policy consultancy work for the government Department of Health. Having worked there for 14 years, I could efficiently deliver policy analysis and updates to support the department, without having to juggle several work streams simultaneously.

As part of the consultancy work, I reviewed the Northern Ireland electronic law repository appraising the interface between housing and healthcare policy to identify relevant legislation and articles. It saved managers, researchers and policy makers hundreds of hours reading and interpreting dozens of documents. At the click of a button the relevant information is there.

As the pandemic began, I was approached by Viva Access, a training company which specialises in disability design courses applied to housing. They needed help to convert their face-to-face courses to being remotely delivered and it proved highly successful and gave me positive focus during the pandemic. It also encouraged me to acquire a whole new range of IT skills.

With the courses covering commonly encountered adaptations, they are solid and practical postgraduate courses for Community OTs and other housing practitioners.

They have now been accredited by Ulster University, which will help to raise the standards of practice in this area.

What else are you involved in now?

I have linked up with Sailability, a group who promote sailing for disabled people in the North West of Northern Ireland and other parts of the world. It has branches all around the country and organises training and competitions.

I am a keen sailor having sailed to various Scottish Islands including the Outer Hebrides and around the West of Ireland.

I have combined my love of sailing and nature with supporting disabled people to get into the water and develop new skills. I have undertaken access studies of the facilities, and I advise on specialised equipment or customed adaptations. I am not just a volunteer, I am also a participant as I have an acquired upper limb disability and I need adjustments and adaptations out on the boats myself, so we learn from each other.

You have mentioned a few role models or people who have inspired or helped you along your journey. Is there anyone else you would like to mention?

David Bass was the Head of the Housing Executive grants service in N. Ireland. He sadly passed away too early. He was a gentle visionary with a highly tuned sense of social justice and he also made a significant contribution to prison reform in Northern Ireland. He was a great inspiration for me and a huge loss as a friend.

Throughout my career I was fortunate to have largely supportive and positive managers and colleagues from a whole variety of professional backgrounds. I learned from every one of them.

Adrian Blythe of Northern Ireland Housing Executive and I also had great synergy, undertaking a range of successful housing design projects together, such as the cost benefit analysis of Lifetime Homes and the inclusive design guide. We brought our complementary perspectives to the table, and I have great respect for his calm, collaborative, problem-solving approach.

Shane Elliott became my successor and he's another colleague with whom I enjoy a very positive working relationship. He also has a strong commitment to and leadership skills for cross-departmental working with a great can-do attitude.

Hazel Winning was my line Manager at the Department of Health and she had a lovely ethos of profiling and publicly celebrating innovation and the achievements of all the Allied Health Professions (AHPs.) I felt this was badly needed to raise the morale and confidence of AHPs often working under severe pressures.

I have also been very impressed with your model Martina, again stepping outside of the norms, moving into a strong family-run business, bringing OT skills into the heart of a highly successful and sophisticated industrial model with worldwide horizons.

What would you say to anyone considering a career in Occupational Therapy?

I think a major attraction of OT as a career is there are so many different areas to work in. You are not tied to any particular one. Whatever your flair or ability there is something to suit everyone. There are many newly developing roles as well. You also have the ability to move around until you find your niche. I moved into several different roles: clinician; researcher; manager; academia and finally government, but there was a constant skill transference taking place, each career move supported by the ones before.

Where would you like to see transformation in the future?

I would like to see more regional evidence-based commissioning of services. It would result in more equality and strategic assessment of need. It should not be a postcode lottery. Limited resources should be fairly targeted to those most in need. There is a major review on assistive technology coming to conclusion. We need to have a more integrated and coordinated approach to the needs assessment and commissioning of those services. This would mean more equality; currently different regions have different budgets for equipment. It is based on the historical patterns of expenditure not based on the needs of the population. So, it needs to be population focused. I think a lot has been achieved through recycling and reusing equipment and there is probably more scope in that area too.

'Being able to move a piece of specialised equipment between NHS health trusts as a regional resource, not necessarily always within the geographical area in which it was originally prescribed.'

This trait keeps arising across public services when people are protecting narrowly defined budgets and not looking at the big picture. We could save a lot of money by smarter use of budgets. The idea of pooled three-year budgets in the future would solve some issues, where resources do not become buried in one sector e.g., the acute hospital.

Further exploration of using remote electronic communications technology to promote work-life balance, productivity and to reduce transport costs and the carbon footprint are needed. I travelled across Northern Ireland for 25 years to deliver my work. Four additional hours a day less with my family. I often lobbied to use remote methods, but it took the COVID-19 pandemic to really bed this in as routine work practice.

Our society has much more to do to process the shock of the pandemic, one almost suspects a collective amnesia about aspects of it, such was the pain.

In certain circumstances I believe long COVID needs to be formally recognised as a disabling condition. This needs to be considered in the long-term planning of our Occupational Therapy services. OTs offer a particularly effective skill set in managing the fatigue, anxiety and social isolation associated with long COVID.

Another major role for OTs is in the prevention of accidents and injuries including to carers. I believe that needs a lot more work. The scale of musculoskeletal injuries is significant and the cost of it is increasing. There is a growing (and ageing) population which needs our help.

What for you is the Power of OT?

It is hard to sum up the Power of OT but when I reflect on my own father, he was a pharmacist, a very practical man who was hardworking and a great provider. As he got older, he suffered from several of the ailments of older age. I remember he was having different health interventions and surgeries; he was in his early 70s when he said one day 'The most important thing in our life is Occupational Therapy. I can see that clearly now.'

He loved the power of purposeful activity. He said 'That is the most important thing to keep me going, it gives me exercise, I need to get a sweat up each day to feel good. I need my golf and attending sports and music events to meet people, it is the biggest thing in my life. As long as I can get out of bed and dress myself I am happy.'

In 2017 cancer, heart disease and a permanently disabling accident entered my life over a three-month period. I was destined not just to know about disability but to personally experience it too. One housing colleague said it was ironic that I would end up with a disability, as if I had some immunity because of my profession!

It was quite a long hard battle to regain the ability to drive, sail and play the violin but when I did, I regained my sense of purpose and joy for living.

I strongly believe purposeful, satisfying activity is right at the heart of the whole profession.

I watched a fascinating television series called 'The Blue Zone' and they looked right across planet earth to see where people live the longest, and the happiest lives. They were finding these pockets of people living to over 100 years of age. They looked at what it was about their lifestyles that gave them such longevity.

There was a lot of overlap but there were also interesting differences with some of the communities they examined. Right at the centre was a sense of purpose, where the whole society was organised to give them a sense of purpose. In a social context the awful blight of loneliness in older age can be broken down by purposeful activity, exercise and social interaction.

'So, to answer the question I thought the Blue Zone really demonstrated the Power of OT. A lot of the underpinning principles and practices of Occupational Therapy contribute to long and happy living.'

Martina's Key Takeaway: As a profession we have come a long way and achieved so much, but there is so much more to do. We should never underestimate our value.

18

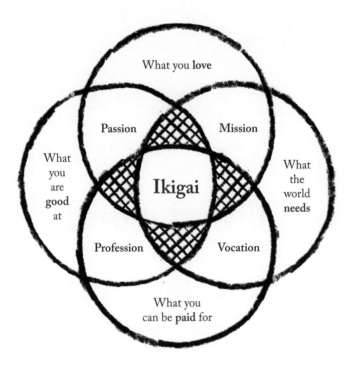

Ikigai (ee-key-guy)

Olivia Tierney

Advanced Practitioner OT in Stroke

Northern Ireland

'Occupational Therapy was something that just matched up with me as a person.'

I could not finish this book on the Power of OT without including my daughter-in-law, Olivia. I first met Olivia when she was 16 years old. My son Ryan brought her home to meet me, she was the first girl he ever took home. She was doing her GCSE's, so I asked her what she planned on doing when she left school. To my amazement she said, 'I am going to be an OT.' Although I was the first OT she had ever actually met, it was not me who influenced her, she already had her heart and mind set on it.

Olivia has been a member of our family since that day but also proved to be a very important member of the Seating Matters team when I needed her most. Olivia qualified in 2012 just when my husband was diagnosed with cancer at age 52. The diagnosis was a huge shock and completely threw me off course. By then I was working full-time in Seating Matters mainly doing training, product evaluation and clinical trials. By this stage Olivia had been around the company and the family for about 5 years. She was very familiar with the therapeutic seating we made and the clinical training, so she stepped straight into my shoes and carried on the work while I took time out to look after James. She proved to be a very capable replacement despite her young age, and she left a lasting impression on many OTs across the world who 10 years later still talk about the training events she delivered with confidence and enthusiasm. Her knowledge was extensive, and her passion was infectious. I am forever grateful to her for taking on this responsibility and giving me that precious time with James.

So Olivia, what is your current role as an OT?

Since 2017 I have worked in an acute stroke ward in one of the main acute hospitals in Northern Ireland. I began my time there as a Specialist Practitioner OT and am now an Advanced Practitioner Occupational Therapist. I currently job share with another OT and together we specialise in stroke assessment and early rehabilitation. We have developed a great team on the ward who are very passionate about stroke care and passionate about the role of OT in early stroke assessment and rehabilitation. We are very committed to advancing our treatment and keeping abreast of new treatments in other hospitals both locally and nationally. An important informant in our role is following the SSNAP protocol* to ensure our patients are receiving the best intervention possible for improved outcomes and that we are measurable alongside other stroke centres.

I have always been passionate about stroke care and it's the area of Occupational Therapy that I always wanted to work in. It is very complex and all-encompassing; the role of the OT is so very important. The brain is the control centre for who we are and everything we do. Our functional ability can be affected in so many ways following a stroke - sometimes in very obvious and observable ways and sometimes in more subtle ways. Patients who have received OT input regularly reflect on their journey after having a stroke and validate the role that the Occupational Therapist had on their recovery.

In Northern Ireland stroke is one of the leading causes of death. Every three hours someone here has a stroke, so it is important that we have OTs in that area who specialise and are at the cutting edge of treatment and intervention.

---

*The SSNAP (Sentinel Stroke National Audit Programme) protocol measures the quality of care provided to stroke patients in the United Kingdom. It assesses various aspects of stroke care, including the time taken for patients to receive treatment, the use of evidence-based interventions, and patient outcomes. The goal is to improve stroke care and outcomes by identifying areas for improvement and promoting best practice.

What does acute OT intervention look like?

In the acute setting the MDT are often likened to first responders. The patient will present to us as a newly diagnosed stroke patient, shattered and traumatised.

We are the first people to pick up the pieces and help them understand what has happened to them and now what needs to happen to try and put them back together. We will look at the very basic things, the 'bread and butter' of OT. Moving from lying to sitting and then getting out of bed is a basic intervention but one of the most important things we do. It can be very challenging depending on the severity of stroke. Unfortunately, for someone who has had a very severe stroke even that act of going from lying in the bed to sitting up at the edge of the bed is a demanding task. Oftentimes, one of our first goals in stroke assessment is to establish sitting tolerance, assess how they sit at the edge of the bed and from there we will progress to transferring into a chair. We then start to build in functional tasks and work with them to participate in getting washed and dressed, regaining independence in feeding, communication, movement, and postural control. We assess cognitive functioning and if we feel someone may be appropriate for home discharge, we assess their ability to manage basic ADLs safely, like making a meal and maintaining a safe environment. We then liaise with our colleagues in the community stroke team who will continue with their rehabilitation when they leave the hospital.

A very important part of our role is to meet with family. When someone has a stroke, it doesn't just affect that person, the family are also distressed. It is very important that the family are involved in the assessment and rehabilitation process and informed of the person's progress after the stroke. We help them understand what's happening to their loved one, what they can do to help and keep them updated and check in with them. We explain what our role is, what goals we are trying to achieve and how they can help be a part of that.

How did you develop your clinical expertise in stroke?

I believe that much of our learning comes from the experience we build up day-to-day working with patients, but I have also been fortunate enough to complete postgraduate courses at Ulster University in Spasticity Management and Neuroplasticity alongside other courses delivered by colleagues. The postgraduate learning helps inform and develop my practice in stroke care and stroke assessment.

This is a very specialised area, it is crucial we understand how the brain functions, the areas of the brain that are affected by the stroke and how this will exhibit in our patients so we can devise the treatment plan quicker and deliver appropriate treatment for the part of the brain and the functions that have been affected. Research and study are a key part of developing confidence to work in the area of stroke assessment.

What triggered your interest in that area of OT?

My interested was ignited in this area of OT when I was in university. During a Neurology lecture we were shown a video of an elderly gentleman who was sitting at a table in a kitchen being asked to butter a piece of bread. All the equipment that he needed was in front of him and in this video the man demonstrated how he heard the instruction but when he went to butter the bread, he picked up a brush from the table to use instead of the knife.

In the next clip it showed us how once again he was asked to butter the piece of bread but this time, he picked up the knife correctly, but he was not able to coordinate the movement to butter the bread. This demonstrated a simple task which was affected so badly by dyspraxia. The point of this lecture was to teach us the difference between ideational dyspraxia and ideomotor dyspraxia. In short, the ideational dyspraxia was not being able to recognise the tool this man needed to complete the job and its correct use, and the ideomotor part of this task was being able to recognise the tool but not being able to implement the motor plan needed to be able to do the job. I found this lecture fascinating, and I knew that working in that area was something that I wanted to do. I was intrigued by the huge impact a brain impairment can have on even the most basic, simple tasks, the small things that we can take for granted. I empathised with these patients and wanted to be part of the solution to help them regain their function and independence. Occupational Therapy plays a key role here as an encourager to reassure the patient that they can get back to their former role or adapt to a new role and the tools we could put in place to assist them.

Tell me about the early years of your career.

One of my first roles as a qualified OT, and even before then, was with Seating Matters. Owing to family circumstances, and the timeliness of my graduating as an OT, I was in a good position to step in and help in a more formal capacity when needed. Through this work, I was very fortunate to be involved in a research project with Ulster University. As a newly qualified OT, I was available and eager to help and learn. Having spent a lot of time working in Seating Matters as a student, I was very familiar with seating assessment and the importance of the provision of correct seating. I also had the opportunity to complete additional postgraduate training at Ulster University in Seating for Complex Disabilities and Pressure Ulcer Prevention and Management which helped inform my practice and guide me in this complex role. The research project was a Knowledge Transfer Partnership (KTP) where I worked alongside the Principal OT who was assigned to the project and the representatives from the University. We worked with them to devise a research plan looking at the impact of sitting on elderly nursing home residents in three local care homes. It was a randomised control trial (RCT) where we assessed the impact of sitting on pressure injuries, falls prevention, oxygen saturation levels, function etc. I was involved in the assessment process, monitoring and data collection and on completion of the trial, a research paper was presented. I had the opportunity to disseminate the results of this at conferences across the world. I also provided training to OTs and other clinical staff across the UK, Ireland and further afield. This gave me the opportunity to increase my confidence at public speaking and presenting, something I love to do.

It was exciting to share that knowledge and to be at the core of changing practice and influencing others. We used the results of the research to influence not only the assessment process but also, we were able to directly impact the design of chairs to improve the outcomes for our patients. It was a valuable part of my career and it demonstrated how my skills as an OT can be used in so many ways from assessment and training to product design.

It was a huge learning curve for me to get straight into that world of specialised seating so early in my career and it has been so beneficial in my roles since. In the acute stroke setting, getting our patients out of bed is one of the first things we do, and it is one of the biggest moments for the patient and the family to see them sitting out of bed for the first time after their stroke. Early intervention is so crucial and marks the first step in the rehab process.

Because of the experience I gained during the research project I am now able to train other members of the team who have not had the same level of experience in postural management and seating. In my health service role, I am a member of the 'practice development group for specialised seating,' where we discuss issues and ideas with each other to ensure we are maintaining high standards of care across the different areas of OT provision.

Another important thing I learned from that time is that you as the OT in any clinical role become the direct link that connects the clients to the equipment they need to use. A product which can be life-changing, which gives them mobility and freedom from being in a bed and gives them back a degree of independence. It's gratifying as an OT that we have this unique role.

'We should never take for granted or minimise the small tasks and how a simple intervention can enable somebody to do that small task, because if we do, we lose the ethos of what OT is.

It's not about the big things. It's not about flashy things. It's about getting the basics and the small things right.'

One of the inherent characteristics of OT is empathy. I think OTs go into that role because they understand how the patient may feel and because they want to help them. I think we are drawn to become OTs because we want to help. It's something that's natural to us.

I think everybody in the wider care team is very good at playing their part and has a very good understanding of what the patient may be going through, but very often it's the OTs that are behind the curtain trying to get the patient moving, functioning or doing everyday tasks. Sometimes that's when they can vent their frustrations. Our experience as OTs helps us empathise with the patients and understand these frustrations.

What attracted you to OT in the first place?

I first found out about OT when I was thirteen. It was at a careers session at school, and I was given a prospectus for Ulster University which has an amazing department for the allied health professions in Northern Ireland. Before I read the prospectus, I had wanted to be a Speech and Language Therapist because I always had an interest in languages. My sister was a Physiotherapist, my mother was a Social Worker and so I was always drawn towards the multidisciplinary team, but I didn't know what an Occupational Therapist was at that time.

Then, when I was perusing the allied health professions section of the prospectus, I discovered Occupational Therapy. I read about it and said to myself 'That's absolutely what I want to do!' That was the decision made there and then. I never diverted from that, there was never any query, and I never second guessed it.

It's very hard to define OT but at the core of it is always helping somebody who has been disadvantaged by illness, injury or disability. Something that they never chose or something that affected them from birth which they had no control over. There was (and is) an empathy in me that wanted to give those people the same chance that anybody else had and for them not to feel excluded from doing things that we take for granted.

'Occupational Therapy was something that just matched up with me as a person.'

My first time to meet an OT was when I was 16. In 2006 I had just met Ryan, my now husband and on our first meeting he asked what I wanted to do when I left school. My response was 'You've probably never heard of this, but I want to be an Occupational Therapist.' He just laughed and said, 'My mother is an OT!'

I had never met any OTs, so I thought that was very interesting. I was fortunate to meet you Martina at such a young age and you taught me about OT and what it involved day to day. I think it's essential for anyone considering a career to get hands-on experience. I was lucky enough to get an inside look into what the role involved, the different ways an OT can work, and it all further strengthened my determination to be an OT.

My earliest experiences as an OT student were helping in The Disability Centre during the summer holidays. I had a range of experiences including office work helping with customer enquiries on the phone, cleaning equipment, loading equipment into the van, going out with you on home visits and seeing assessments with clients. I paid attention to how you communicated with clients and other clinicians - it was an invaluable learning experience.

This was one of the best introductions anyone could have gotten into OT because you had set up on your own business to better meet patient needs. I found it a really inspiring story. You overcame your concerns about becoming an OT outside of the health service and that was an important lesson for me. To not be afraid of trying new things and taking a risk.

When you have a good mentor and exposure to different kinds of working then it gives you confidence to know that you can use your training to create a new role for yourself in a new service which can benefit patients. I believe a person should never feel any less of an OT because you're not working directly in the health service. Private practice can work to complement and support other traditional positions.

What do you do to make OT relevant in your work?

I always keep my OT hat on: selfcare, productivity and leisure. I learned this from one of my practice educators on a placement and it has stayed with me ever since.

'Keep the basics in mind and put the patient at the centre of everything you do.'

I think historically it has been difficult to define the OT role because it can look very different depending on the individual and their area of work. However, as the OT you should always know your role and have confidence in what you are doing.

I like to start with why. Why am I here? What can we achieve together? It is important to remember that 'What you measure improves,' so you must know what you are trying to achieve for each person and monitor and reevaluate regularly. This helps ensure you are achieving the desired outcomes and making a difference to that person's life.

Tell me about a memorable experience you've had with a patient.

We had a young patient on the ward with a very significant stroke which was life changing. She had an extended period as an inpatient away from her family, having only one visit per day as she had been quite unwell. Her language and motor function had been severely affected by the stroke. She had difficulty communicating her needs. We observed that her mood became very low, and she wasn't engaging with us. It was difficult to determine what she wanted, and it was becoming difficult to plan treatment sessions which engaged her, but I took a moment to think 'What if this was me... what would make me feel better?'

Up to this point she had only had bed baths. So, I asked her 'Would you like a shower?' She nodded a strong yes! This wasn't revolutionary treatment, it wasn't groundbreaking, but I identified the one thing that would make her feel better. Some people might say that you're doing the Nurse's job, but I don't think the role of the OT stops and the Nurse's begins. We should not be afraid to move across the boundaries if that's what is needed at that time for the good of the patient.

Helping her shower enabled us to build rapport, we encouraged her to participate in her own rehabilitation and we gained her trust as a team who cared about her wellbeing. It improved her mood and her motivation. When the water was splashing over her, you could see the relief on her face, this was something she identified with from her old life, just a very simple basic act of washing. We washed her hair and shaved her legs and as a young female this was so important for her self-image and how she felt about herself. It gave her back self-respect and dignity, she started to regain a bit of herself in that moment.

What would you say to an OT student or someone who is considering a career in OT?

I don't think there's anything more effective I could say to them than 'Go and see!'

Go to the workplace and observe what it is that you'll be doing.' It's not something that you take lightly. If you pursue the career of an OT, you will have a very important role that will impact a lot of people at very pivotal and vulnerable moments of their life so you need to have a well-rounded idea of what the profession involves and the skills you need to be an effective OT.

Then, after qualification you should never stop learning. Never think you know enough. Don't get complacent. I would also say to students and young graduates don't be afraid to work outside the traditional roles. These new roles help to strengthen and build up the reputation of our profession.

I think OTs can have an influential role in industry in terms of research, product development and education. My experience working with manufacturers and researchers was very enriching and empowering in that you could sit slightly outside the traditional roles, but you have the power to directly influence the clinicians by providing research and evidence to justify their clinical interventions. OTs have the clinical knowledge and skills to impact and influence product design and innovation, it's an important role for OTs now and in the future.

There is also scope for more OTs to become involved in vocational rehabilitation and workplace adjustments to get people into the workplace or maintaining them in the workplace. Our strength is in activity analysis, we stage tasks and simplify activities to enable the person to adapt to a new job or return to a former job. OT skills could be used in manufacturing processes to create flow and lessen the burden on employees whether it is someone returning to work following an illness or injury or as a preventative measure to reduce injuries in the workplace.

'Happy and successful OTs help make happy and successful patients.'

If you could influence transformation in one area of OT, what would it be?

I would love to see more OTs finding an area they are very passionate about and excelling in that area early in their career. Oftentimes the recruitment process compels new recruits to take up posts which may not be an area of their choice and limits their options.

What is the Power of OT?

I believe you need enthusiasm for your job to give it your best. Patients benefit most from OTs who are passionate and dedicated to their area of work and the profession is driven by passionate OTs.

There's a Japanese philosophy which I have always loved called 'Ikigai.'

ikigai
[ee-key-guy] *noun*

A Japanese concept that combines the terms iki, meaning "alive" or "life," and gai, meaning "benefit" or "worth."

When combined, these terms mean 'That which gives your life worth, meaning, or purpose.'

In short, it is the 'sweet spot' between something you love (your passion,) what the world needs (your mission,) what you are good at (your vocation,) and what you can get paid for (your profession.)

I think Ikigai sums up the Power of Occupational Therapy really well, especially when you find your 'sweet spot' in the profession.

Martina's Key Takeaway: Find your 'sweet spot.'

Conclusion

Writing this book, reflecting on my own career and interviewing the dedicated and inspiring OTs from around the world has energised me about my profession. It has motivated me to want to start over again and show the world the Power of OT. It is my hope that this book will do that for the reader. Throughout the interviews all the OTs talked about the importance of continual learning. Continual education and research benefits everyone. It instils more confidence in the therapist about their role and their intervention, it elevates the role of OT among other professionals but most importantly the patient/client benefits from the enhanced expertise of the OT. If you want to transform your profession and the impact you can have on your patient, continual learning is essential. It is said that Michelangelo's last words at the age of 87 were 'Ancora imparo' which means 'I am still learning.' We must always continue to learn and advance our practice.

At the heart of all the interviews were emotional and heartfelt stories about the patients and clients. It demonstrated clearly that for OTs the patient is at the heart of everything we do. Many of the stories were about the ordinary everyday things that mattered to the patient. Whether it was being able to hold a cigarette independently, planting sunflowers, looking after chickens, having a shower or being able to sit up in a chair and take a sip of water without assistance, it was often the simple things that mattered most to the patient. As OTs we should never lose sight of the simple things. It may seem menial to others but to the patient it means everything, and we should be proud of our intervention which enables and empowers our patient to do the everyday tasks. We make the difficult tasks achievable for the patient through activity analysis, equipment provision, adaptation or therapeutic intervention.

I was very proud to hear how many of the OTs who contributed to the book have transformed the profession in various ways and have thereby transformed the lives of the patients. Many have lobbied government and successfully changed legislation. Others have carried out research to provide evidence for the need to change the status quo, and to advance their practice for the benefit of the patient while others are involved in educating and invigorating the next generation of OTs.

'Leave it Better Than You Found it.'

This book has shown examples of OTs who were previously employed in different jobs retraining as OTs when they saw the benefit or the need for Occupational Therapy. We also touched on the apprenticeship pathway to OT and the skills of the Occupational Therapy Assistant which sometimes go unnoticed but are making a massive contribution to the profession. It is important that both these opportunities are further explored so we can maximise the skills that exist in the workforce and use them to benefit the Occupational Therapy profession. OT is unique as it offers so many opportunities both within a public sector job or in the private sector. OTs can work in either or both, as one OT said, 'We are limited only by our imagination. Many OTs have a portfolio career where they can have a variety of experiences with each experience complementing the other.'

Some of the OTs I spoke to entered the profession by accident, others were influenced by personal experiences, and some knew from early in their education that OT was their vocation, but all the OTs said they would do it all over again and many, including myself, felt that we were born to be Occupation Therapists. Individually and collectively, we have the power to transform the world of healthcare and in doing so transform the world of the patients and clients who need us most.

In 2021 we were honoured to have the Patron of the RCOT, HRH The Princess Royal visit the Seating Matters factory. She toured the manufacturing facility and expressed great knowledge of and interest in our products. She also connected very accurately the link between the Occupational Therapy values and the clinical designs of our chairs. On leaving she congratulated us on 'Our outstanding product, brought about by an incredibly innovative team.' It was the icing on the cake for me as an Occupational Therapist to be recognised by her as someone who is making a difference in the lives of our most vulnerable patients.

'Leave it Better Than You Found it' is one of the guiding principles of Seating Matters. One of our goals is to leave each person better than we found them, whether it's a patient, a family member, an employee or a visitor we hope they feel better after we have left them or they have left us.

My vision is also to leave the profession of Occupational Therapy better than I found it and with your help together we can achieve that for the benefit of the next generation of Occupational Therapists. Let's spread the word on the Power of OT.

'The meaning of life is to find your gift.
The purpose of life is to give it away.'

Further Reading

The Clinician's Seating Handbook

The Clinician's Seating Handbook is used in academia, in clinical practice and with caregivers around the world to guide their practices around specialist seating and contains;

- Practical tips on cultivating a 24 hour package of care
- Your guide for supporting various spinal presentations
- A guide to seating plus-size and paediatric patients
- Information on the new staging guidelines for pressure injuries
- Detailed patient case studies

To order your copy visit **seatingmatters.com**

Scan here

The Stairway of My Life

The Stairway of My Life is a memoir with a message. It takes us through Martina's life from a child helping on the farm, to training to become an Occupational Therapist and setting up her own business, which became a global success.

To find out more visit **martinatierney.com**

Scan here